ATLAS

For Churchill Livingstone

Publisher: Timothy Horne
Project Editors: Barbara Simmons, Janice Urquhart
Copy Editor: Joanna Smith
Project Controller: Nancy Arnott
Design & Electronic Page Make-up: Charles Simpson
Promotions Executive: Duncan Jones

ANATOMY: A DISSECTION MANUAL AND ATLAS

S. JACOB

MBBS MS (Anatomy)
Lecturer in Anatomy and Cell Biology
Department of Biomedical Science
University of Sheffield

Dissections by
David J. Hinchliffe MIAS

Photography by
Mick A. Turton

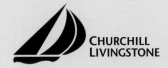

CHURCHILL LIVINGSTONE

NEW YORK EDINBURGH LONDON MADRID
MELBOURNE SAN FRANCISCO AND TOKYO 1996

CHURCHILL LIVINGSTONE
Medical Division of Pearson Professional Limited

Distributed in the United States of America by Churchill
Livingstone Inc., 650 Avenue of the Americas, New York,
N.Y. 10011, and by associated companies, branches and
representatives throughout the world.

First published 1996

ISBN 0 443 04852 5

British Library Cataloguing in Publication Data
A catalogue record for this book is available from the
British Library

Library of Congress Cataloging in Publication Data
A Catalog record for this book is available from the
Library of Congress

The
publisher's
policy is to use
**paper manufactured
from sustainable forests**

Printed in Hong Kong

Contents

Preface

The best way of learning Anatomy is by dissection. It allows 3-dimensional examination of the various parts of the body. This book, intended for students learning gross anatomy for the first time, deals with the dissection of the most important features of the human body. The text contains dissection instruction with concise descriptions of structures exposed and a brief account of their clinical application. This is balanced with numerous colour illustrations, most of them photographs of dissections.

In my experience, many students, do not like to read lengthy descriptions given in dissection manuals, even if they are given time to do this in the dissecting room. Dissection laboratories are usually crowded, noisy and on the whole do not present a congenial atmosphere for reading and studying detailed descriptive anatomy. With this in mind I have restricted the background text to bare essentials hoping that further details will be read from textbooks at a later stage. However, as the majority of students learning Anatomy for the first time are medical students the clinical application of the part being dissected is emphasised in the text to illustrate the relevance of the subject to the medical profession. The illustrations presented here should help the student during dissection as well as self-study and revision.

In planning this book, I have taken into account the time constraint affecting modern Anatomy courses. It attempts to cover only the most important features of each topic. Though this is not a complete source book of Anatomy, it is hoped that it will encourage the student to pursue dissection with interest and enthusiasm.

I wish to thank the production team at Churchill Livingstone for the constant encouragement and practical help throughout the preparation of this book. I am also greatly indebted to Mr David Hinchliffe for producing the excellent dissections, Mr Michael Turton for his exceptional expertise in photography, Professor A. Angel, Chairman of the Department and Mr Ivan Dart, Laboratory Manager, for providing the facilities in the Department of Biomedical Science, University of Sheffield.

Sheffield   *S. Jacob*
1996

INTRODUCTION

1

Dissection

Anatomy is the study of the structure of the body. The word is derived from the Greek word *anat'ome* which means to cut up. The Latin equivalent of this is *dissecare* from which the word dissection has derived.

Dissection of a cadaver is an *active learning* process by which the three dimensional architecture of the human body is appreciated. It will allow the student to appreciate the way the structures are packaged in the body, the depth at which they lie and also their size and relationship to one another. Dissection facilitates interactive learning among a small group of students around a table. It teaches team work, imparts academic discipline and provides confidence in one's own ability.

THE VOCABULARY OF ANATOMY

Anatomy has a highly specialised vocabulary, mostly derived from Greek or Latin. The *anatomical position*, about which the anatomical relations of structures are described, is that in which the person stands erect, arms by the sides, palms of the hands facing forwards (Fig. 1.1). Structures in front are termed *anterior* and those behind, *posterior*. Structures above are *superior* and those below, *inferior*. Structures nearer the midline of the body are *medial* and those away from the midline, *lateral*. Structures nearer to the surface are *superficial* and those further from the surface are deep. In

the limbs, the term *proximal* is used to describe structures nearer to the trunk and *distal* for those away from the trunk. A *sagittal plane* passes vertically anteroposteriorly through the body and the *coronal plane* is at right angles to the sagittal plane (Fig. 1.1).

Movements (Fig. 1.2). Movement in the coronal plane away from the midsagittal plane is called *abduction*, return towards the midsagittal plane is *adduction*. Bending of any part in the sagittal plane is *flexion* and straightening is *extension*. *Rotation* occurs around a vertical axis. It may be medial rotation, towards the midline or *lateral*, away from it.

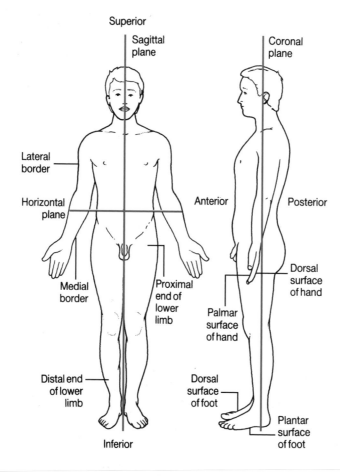

Fig. 1.1 **The anatomical position**

ABOUT THIS BOOK

In this book the dissection methods are presented on a regional basis starting with the upper limb, followed by thorax, abdomen, lower limb and finally the head and neck. Though this order is preferred it can be dissected in any order provided slight alterations are made by the instructor. The drastic reduction of time available for dissection has been taken into account in preparation of this dissection manual. What is described in each chapter can be dissected in a two hour dissection period. Thus about 96 hours are required to dissect the whole body using this book.

Each chapter of the book contains dissection instructions and background text with detailed illustrations consisting of photographs of dissections and line drawings. The text apart from brief description of the relevant parts also contains osteology, surface anatomy and clinical anatomy.

Osteology. This is the study of bones and is an important part of gross anatomy. Only the bare essentials are mentioned in each chapter. Details should be learned by using a textbook.

Surface anatomy. This is the art of projecting on to the surface the underlying structures. Many definitive elements of the living body can be easily identified on the surface. Examine each other and learn from it. Eventually it is the living subjects that many students will deal with as professionals. Ignorance of this part of anatomy will be a serious handicap for a medical student during physical examination of a patient!

Clinical anatomy. Of all the basic science courses that a medical student takes, none are more directly related to their professional practice than is gross anatomy and its application. The knowledge of clinical applications of anatomy enlivens anatomy for science students as well. In this book clinical anatomy is presented, in each chapter, as separate paragraphs with a different colour coding.

HOW TO DISSECT

Make the best use of the time allowed for dissection. Read about the area to be dissected beforehand. Follow the instructions. Do not dig around blindly. Look at the illustrations frequently to see what you are supposed to see.
Always try to demonstrate structures as clearly as possible. 'Clean' the structures by removing fat, connective tissue and small veins.

You do not need many instruments to dissect. Scalpels are required for skin reflection. Two pairs of forceps, a large one and a small one, are useful for cleaning structures. Hold the structure using the large forceps and clean with the small one. Avoid damaging structures by employing the use of *blunt dissection*. This applies in surgery too. Use your fingers, handle of the scalpel or a pair of forceps to separate and clean structures. Do not cut them with sharp instruments.

You get out of a dissection class exactly in proportion to what you put into it — no more and no less. It is always a privilege to have the opportunity to dissect a human body. The cadaver you dissect is the best textbook of anatomy available. Enjoy its study.

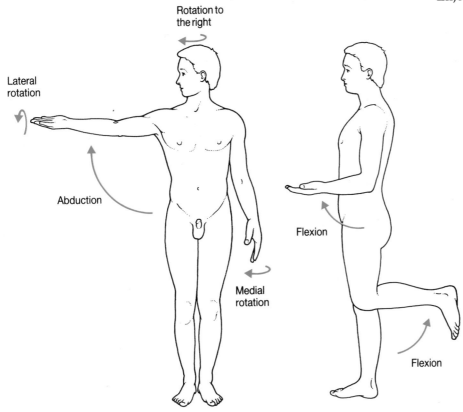

Fig. 1.2 **Movements of the head and limbs**

THE UPPER LIMB

2

The pectoral region

Osteology

Refer to Figure 2.1 and identify the following on the articulated skeleton:

- clavicle
- acromial process of the scapula
- coracoid process of the scapula
- sternum
- jugular notch
- xiphoid process of the sternum
- humerus.

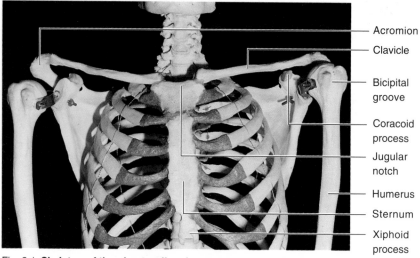

Fig. 2.1 **Skeleton of the chest wall and upper arm — anterior view**

Surface anatomy

Refer to Figure 2.2 and identify the following on your partner:

- clavicle
- sternum
- jugular notch
- xiphoid process of the sternum
- sternoclavicular joint
- acromial process of the scapula
- areola and nipple
- lower costal margin.

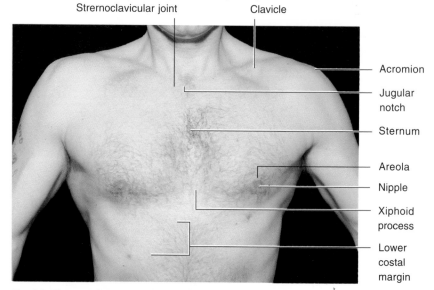

Fig. 2.2 **Chest and upper arm — anterior view**

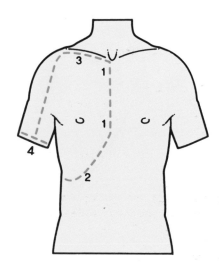

Fig. 2.3 **Incision lines**

Skin reflection

Make the following skin incisions (Fig. 2.3):

1. a midline incision extending from the jugular notch to the xiphoid process
2. an incision along the lower costal margin
3. an incision along the clavicle from the jugular notch to the acromial process extending downwards to the middle of the arm
4. a circular one around the arm from the lower end of the last incision.

Reflect the skin laterally from the midline. As you do so look for:

- the cutaneous nerves and vessels emerging from the intercostal spaces through the overlying muscles
- the lactiferous ducts of the mammary gland opening into the nipple.

Remove the mammary gland, noting that it is not attached to the deep fascia over the pectoralis major muscle.

Remove the remaining superficial fascia and the deep fascia and expose and clean the pectoralis major muscle fully (Fig. 2.4).

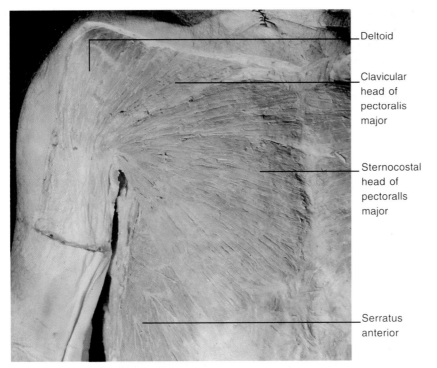

Deltoid

Clavicular head of pectoralis major

Sternocostal head of pectoralis major

Serratus anterior

Fig. 2.4 **Pectoralis major muscle**

PECTORALIS MAJOR

Origin. The medial third of the clavicle (clavicular head) and the sternum and costal cartilages (sternocostal head).

Insertion. The lateral lip of the bicipital groove on the shaft of the humerus.

Action. The sternocostal fibres adduct and rotate the humerus medially at the shoulder joint. The clavicular fibres flex the humerus.

Nerve supply. The lateral and medial pectoral nerves.

> Identify *deltoid*, which is the large muscle covering the shoulder region. The *cephalic vein*, a superficial vein of the arm, may be seen in the groove between deltoid and pectoralis major.

Reflection of the pectoralis major

> Detach the clavicular head of the muscle from the clavicle and reflect it carefully towards the arm. Note the lateral pectoral nerve entering the deep surface of the muscle.
>
> Detach the sternocostal head from its origin and reflect it laterally. The medial pectoral nerve will now be seen entering its deep surface after piercing the underlying pectoralis minor.
>
> Examine the pectoralis minor (Fig. 2.5).

PECTORALIS MINOR

Origin. Third to fifth (often second to fourth) ribs.

Insertion. The coracoid process of the scapula.

Action. Pectoralis minor draws the scapula (hence the arm) forwards — protraction of the shoulder. It can also depress the shoulder.

Nerve supply. Medial pectoral nerve.

> Verify that the anterior wall of the axilla (armpit) is formed throughout by pectoralis major and that it is reinforced in its middle by the pectoralis minor muscle.

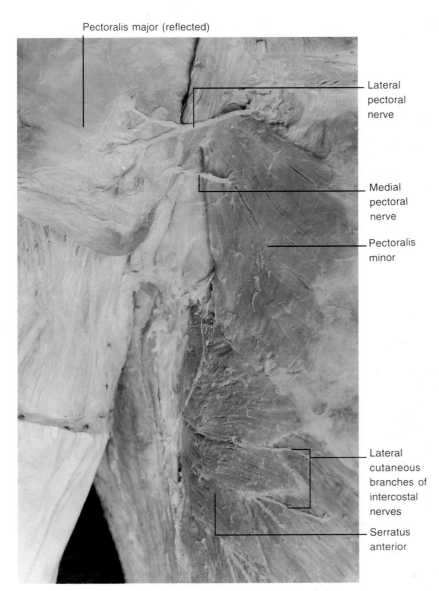

Pectoralis major (reflected)

Lateral pectoral nerve

Medial pectoral nerve

Pectoralis minor

Lateral cutaneous branches of intercostal nerves

Serratus anterior

Fig. 2.5 **Structures seen after reflection of pectoralis major**

3

The back of the trunk

Osteology

Refer to Figure 3.1 and identify the following on the articulated skeleton:

- external occipital protuberance on the skull
- mastoid process
- spinous process of the seventh cervical vertebra (the most prominent spinous process at the nape of the neck)
- spinous processes of thoracic vertebrae
- spine of the scapula continuing as the acromial process
- medial and lateral margins of the scapula
- sacrum and iliac crest.

Surface anatomy

Identify the bony points listed above on your partner.

Skin reflection

Turn the cadaver over so that it lies face downwards. Make the following incisions:

1. a vertical incision from the external occipital protuberance to the sacrum
2. a transverse incision from the external occipital protuberance laterally to the mastoid process
3. a transverse incision from the spinous process of the seventh thoracic vertebra to the acromial process
4. a curved incision along the iliac crest
5. a transverse incision midway between 3 and 4.

Reflect the skin and the superficial fascia.

Refer to Figure 3.2 and clean the *trapezius* and the *latissimus dorsi*. The cutaneous nerves, which emerge near the midline in series, are the dorsal rami of the spinal nerves.

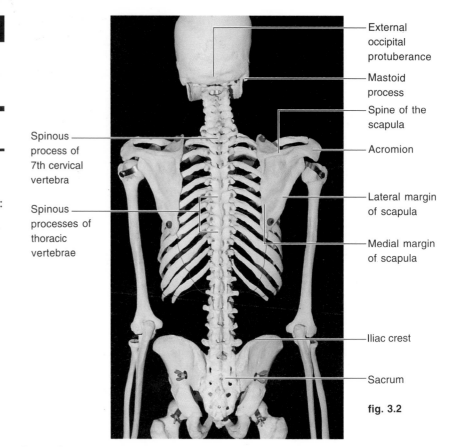

fig. 3.2

Fig. 3.1 **Skeleton of the trunk and upper limb seen from the back**

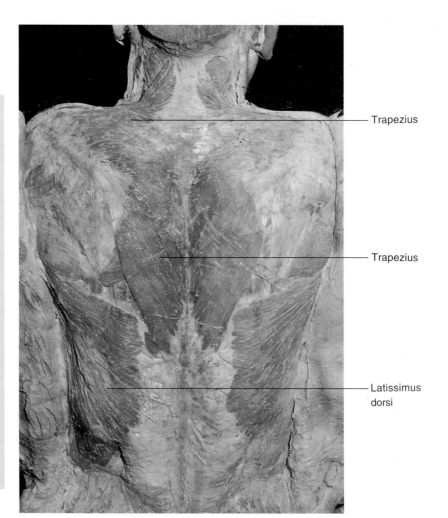

Fig. 3.2 **Superficial muscles of the back**

TRAPEZIUS

Origin
- External occipital protuberance and the superior nuchal line
- Ligamentum nuchae — fibro-elastic tissue connecting the muscle to the spines of the cervical vertebrae
- Spinous processes of the seventh cervical to the twelfth thoracic vertebrae.

Insertion
- Upper fibres to the lateral part of clavicle
- Middle fibres to the acromion
- Lower fibres to the spine of the scapula.

Action. Trapezius rotates the scapula so that the glenoid cavity faces upwards. This action is important for raising the arm above the level of the shoulder. The shoulder is elevated by the upper fibres (as in shrugging the shoulder).

Nerve supply. Spinal part of the accessory nerve.

Reflection of trapezius

Insert the handle of the scalpel under the lateral border and free the muscle from the underlying structures.

Detach the muscle from its origin by a vertical incision.

Reflect the muscle laterally taking extreme care that you are reflecting only trapezius (it is a very thin muscle).

Reflect the muscle fully by detaching it from its insertion to the spine of the scapula and acromion and leave it attached to the clavicle. As you do so, dissect out the accessory nerve accompanied by vessels in the fascia on the deep surface of the muscle (Fig. 3.3).

LATISSIMUS DORSI (Fig. 3.2)

Origin
- Spinous processes of the lower six thoracic vertebrae
- Thoracolumbar fascia that covers the deep muscles of the back
- Posterior part of the outer lip of the iliac crest.

The muscle sweeps around the side of the body to be inserted into the humerus.

Insertion. The bicipital groove of the humerus. The insertion may be verified later.

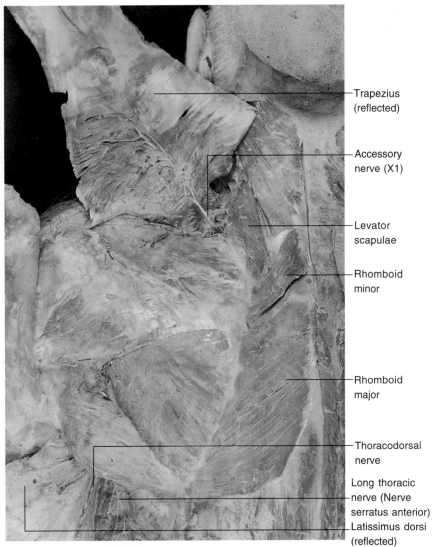

Fig. 3.3 **Structures seen after reflection of the (left side) trapezius and latissimus dorsi**

Trapezius (reflected)

Accessory nerve (X1)

Levator scapulae

Rhomboid minor

Rhomboid major

Thoracodorsal nerve

Long thoracic nerve (Nerve serratus anterior)

Latissimus dorsi (reflected)

Action. The extension, medial rotation and adduction of the shoulder. If the insertion is fixed, it can be used to raise the trunk as in climbing.

Nerve supply. Thoracodorsal nerve.

Reflection of the latissimus dorsi

Cut across the muscle about 5 cm from the midline, after separating it from the underlying structures.

Reflect the lateral half towards the axilla and dissect out the thoraco-dorsal nerve deep to the muscle (the blood vessels accompanying the nerve will act as a guide). The muscle exposed by the reflection of the latissimus dorsi is the lower part of the serratus anterior.

Try and expose the long thoracic nerve supplying the muscle by

referring to Figure 3.3.

Study the levator scapulae, rhomboid minor and rhomboid major exposed by the reflection of trapezius. They are inserted into the medial border of the scapula (Fig. 3.3). Levator scapulae takes origin from the transverse processes and the rhomboids from the spinous pro-cesses of the vertebrae.

Finally, detach the rhomboids (not levator scapulae) from their origins and reflect them laterally.

4

The posterior triangle

The posterior triangle, or the side of the neck, contains the proximal parts of the brachial plexus of nerves supplying the upper limb. Dissection of this part of the neck, followed by dissection of the axilla, will enable you to visualise this complex network of nerves in its entirety.

Surface anatomy

Refer to Figure 4.1 and identify on your partner:

- sternocleidomastoid
- trapezius muscle
- middle part of the clavicle bounding the posterior triangle.

Skin reflection

Extend the skin reflection already done to expose trapezius forward up to the anterior border of the sternomastoid. This should be done carefully without damaging the platysma muscle and the external jugular vein which lie immediately beneath the skin in the superficial fascia.

EXTERNAL JUGULAR VEIN (Fig 4.2)

Reflect platysma carefully and you may see the external jugular vein which drains the scalp and face.

The external jugular vein lies superficial to sternomastoid, but in the lower part of the posterior triangle pierces the deep fascia and drains into the subclavian vein. It is prone to many variations and its size is inversely proportional to the size of other neck veins.

Surface anatomy

Ask your partner to blow with his or her nose and mouth closed (Valsalva manoeuvre) to increase the intra-thoracic pressure. The distended external jugular vein will be seen extending from the angle of the lower jaw to the middle of the clavicle.

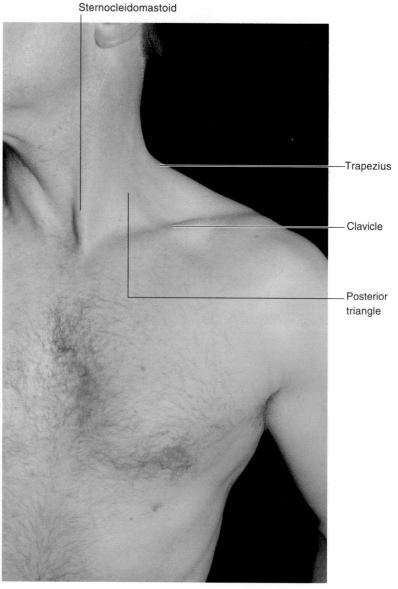

Fig. 4.1 **Boundaries of the (left side) posterior triangle**

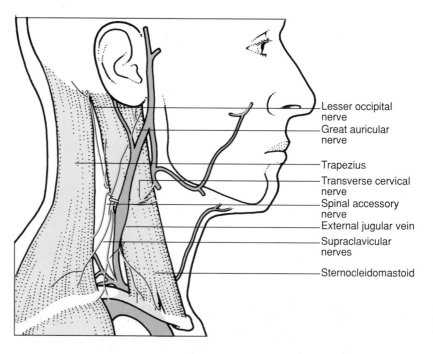

Fig. 4.2 **Superficial structures in the (right side) posterior triangle**

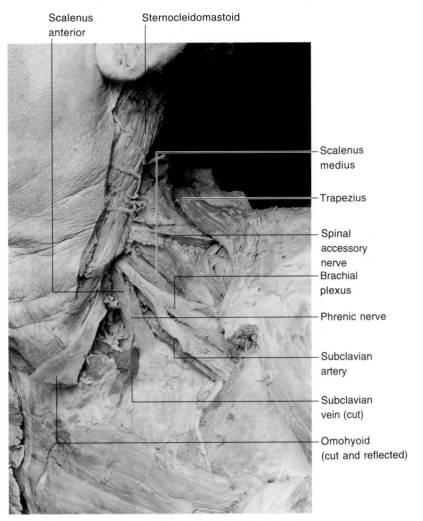

Scalenus anterior Sternocleidomastoid

Scalenus medius

Trapezius

Spinal accessory nerve

Brachial plexus

Phrenic nerve

Subclavian artery

Subclavian vein (cut)

Omohyoid (cut and reflected)

Fig. 4.3 **Deep structures in the (left side) posterior triangle**

OMOHYOID MUSCLE

Identify a slender muscle crossing the lower part of the triangle obliquely. This is omohyoid which is one of the infrahyoid muscles and will be described later (p.135).

Cut the muscle at its lower end and reflect it medially.

Removal of the clavicle

Using a bone-saw, make two cuts on the clavicle, one at the posterior border of sternomastoid and the other at the anterior border of trapezius. It will be easier to cut the bone if the soft tissues are removed from it beforehand.

Use a bone forceps to remove the middle portion of clavicle.

BRACHIAL PLEXUS, SUBCLAVIAN ARTERY SUBCLAVIAN VEIN AND THE PHRENIC NERVE (Fig. 4.3)

Removal of the clavicle will expose a portion of the first rib and the two muscles attached to it: *scalenus anterior* and *scalenus medius*. This area can be exposed more clearly if the clavicular head of sternocleidomastoid is also reflected. The brachial plexus and the subclavian artery lie between the scalene muscles.

Separate the artery from the brachial plexus. Note that the *subclavian artery* crosses *behind* scalenus anterior.

Clean the *subclavian vein* crossing *in front* of scalenus anterior.

Carefully remove the subclavian vein and its tributaries to get a better exposure of the subclavian artery and the brachial plexus.

The *phrenic nerve* also lies in front of scalenus anterior and crosses it obliquely from its lateral to its medial border (Fig. 4.3). Identify and clean the nerve.

Finally, separate the components of the brachial plexus. You will be able to identify the *upper, middle* and *lower trunks* of the plexus stacked one on top of the other.

Clean the vein, note its course and remove it and its tributaries.

anterior border of the trapezius about 5 cm above the clavicle.

✳ The spinal accessory nerve, because of its superficial position, can be damaged in the posterior triangle. The trapezius muscle will be paralysed, resulting in inability to lift the arm above the level of the shoulder (p.9).

STERNOCLEIDOMASTOID

Origin. By two heads from the manubrium of the sternum and the clavicle.

Insertion. The mastoid process and superior nuchal line.

Action. Sternocleidomastoid turns the head to the opposite side.

Nerve supply. Spinal accessory nerve.

SPINAL ACCESSORY NERVE (Figs 4.2 and 4.3)

Find the accessory nerve supplying the trapezius muscle. It can be easily traced into the triangle if it is already identified under the trapezius (Fig. 4.3).

Surface marking. The nerve can be marked on the surface by drawing a line connecting a point just above the middle of the posterior border of the sternomastoid to a point on the

Cervical plexus

Cutaneous branches of this plexus supply the skin of the neck, the shoulder and pectoral regions. They are:

- Great auricular nerve (C2, C3)
- Lesser occipital nerve (C2)
- Transverse cervical nerve (C2, C3)
- Supraclavicular nerves (C3, C4).

Try to find some of these branches (Fig 4.2). The *phrenic nerve* (C3, C4, C5) supplying the diaphragm and the inferior root of the *ansa cervicalis* for the infrahyoid muscles are also branches of the cervical plexus and will be dissected later.

5

The axilla

The axilla or the armpit is the space between the trunk and the upper arm. It is pyramidal in shape and its boundaries are:

- *anterior wall* — the pectoralis major and pectoralis minor muscles
- *posterior wall* — the subscapularis, teres major and latissimus dorsi muscles
- *lateral wall* — the upper end of the humerus with the biceps brachii and the coracobrachialis muscles
- *medial wall* — the serratus anterior muscle covering the ribs and intercostal spaces
- *apex* — formed by the first rib medially with the clavicle in front and the scapula behind. It is the channel of communication between the posterior triangle and the axilla
- *base* — skin and deep fascia extending between the chest wall and the arm.

SURFACE ANATOMY

Abduct your partner's arm slightly and feel the boundaries of the axilla. Feel the bones bounding its apex by deep palpation.
The axilla contains:

- fat and lymph nodes
- axillary artery and vein
- brachial plexus.

✳ The lymph nodes in the axilla are of tremendous clinical importance as they drain the mammary gland. Carcinoma of the breast can spread into these lymph nodes. Axillary lymph nodes drain not only the lymphatics of the breast, but also those of the pectoral region, upper abdominal wall and the upper limb.

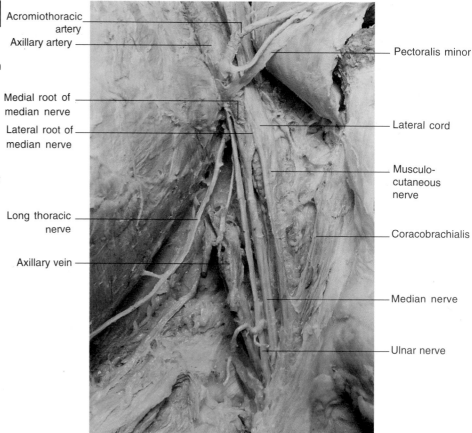

Fig. 5.1 **Dissection of the (left side) axilla**

Acromiothoracic artery
Axillary artery
Medial root of median nerve
Lateral root of median nerve
Long thoracic nerve
Axillary vein

Pectoralis minor
Lateral cord
Musculo-cutaneous nerve
Coracobrachialis
Median nerve
Ulnar nerve

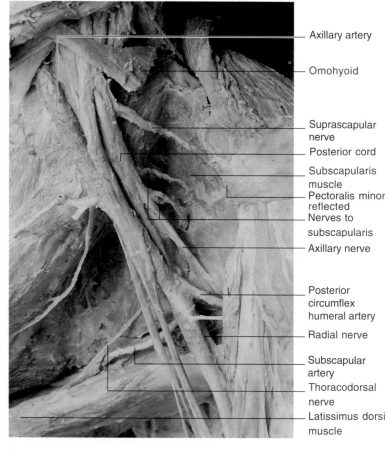

Axillary artery
Omohyoid
Suprascapular nerve
Posterior cord
Subscapularis muscle
Pectoralis minor reflected
Nerves to subscapularis
Axillary nerve
Posterior circumflex humeral artery
Radial nerve
Subscapular artery
Thoracodorsal nerve
Latissimus dorsi muscle

Fig. 5.2 **Deep dissection of the (left side) axilla.** The axillary artery and the lateral and medial cords have been pushed medially to show the posterior cord and its branches

Dissection of the axilla

Incise the pectoralis minor from its origin and reflect it laterally. This will expose the contents more fully. By blunt dissection with fingers and forceps remove carefully the fat and lymph nodes and expose the axillary artery and vein and the lower parts of the brachial plexus (Fig. 5.1). You will notice that these are covered by a fascial sheath — the *axillary sheath* — which is a prolongation of the fascia covering the muscles in the posterior triangle (the prevertebral fascia). Remove the sheath making sure that you do not cut the nerves and the branches of the axillary artery. Having noted the position of the axillary vein medial to the artery remove the vein and its tributaries to get a better exposure of the artery and the brachial plexus.

Identify the part of the axillary artery lying deep to the pectoralis minor. Lift up the lateral cord of the brachial plexus lying lateral to this part of the artery (Fig. 5.1) and using a forceps clean its branches. The *musculo-cutaneous nerve* will be seen entering the coracobrachialis muscle. Another major branch is the lateral root of the median nerve. Identify the median nerve and its medial and lateral roots. These three form the shape of the letter 'M'. Trace the medial root of the median nerve upwards and identify the medial cord lying medial to the axillary artery. Trace the branches of the medial cord. All of them lie medial to the artery. The medial cutaneous nerve of the forearm is superficial to the larger *ulnar nerve*. The medial cutaneous nerve of the arm lies further medially. It may be replaced by the *intercostobrachial nerve* which is a branch of the second intercostal nerve. The importance of the intercosto-brachial nerve is that it is the only nerve supplying the upper limb without passing through the brachial plexus.

Retract the axillary artery to one side and identify the posterior cord behind it (Fig. 5.2). Trace its branches. The *axillary nerve* leaves the axilla winding round the surgical neck of the humerus, passing below the shoulder joint. It is accompanied by the posterior circumflex humeral branch of the axillary artery. *The nerve may be paralysed in dislocation of the shoulder joint as well as in a fracture of the surgical neck of the humerus.* The thoracodorsal nerve lies in the loose areolar tissue in front of the subscapularis muscle and can be traced to the latissimus dorsi muscle. The muscle on which the posterior cord lies is the subscapularis. Trace two or three nerves entering the subscapularis from the posterior cord. Clean the continuation of the posterior cord. This is the *radial nerve* which will supply the extensor muscles in the arm and forearm.

Axillary artery (Fig. 5.3)

The axillary artery is a continuation of the subclavian artery and it extends from the outer border of the first rib to the lower border of the teres major from where it continues as the brachial artery. For descriptive purposes it can be divided into three parts by the pectoralis minor. The part above the muscle is the *first* part, the part underneath the *second* and the part below the *third* part. The three cords of the brachial plexus are arranged around the second part of the artery in the following manner (Fig. 5.3):

- lateral cord — lateral to the artery
- medial cord — medial to the artery
- posterior cord — posterior to the artery.

Note that the three cords are named after their relation to the second part of the artery.

The axillary vein is medial to the artery separated from it for most of its course by the medial cord and its branches.

Clean the axillary artery and its branches. The *acromiothoracic, lateral thoracic, posterior circumflex humeral* and the *subscapular arteries* are big branches and should be cleaned without damaging the adjoining nerves (Figs 5.1 & 5.2).

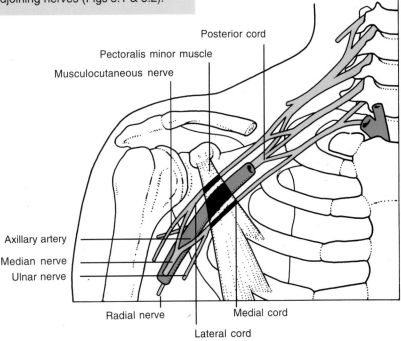

Fig.5.3 **The structures related to the (right side) axillary artery**

Brachial plexus (Figs 5.3 & 5.4)

The brachial plexus innervates the upper limb. It is described as having:

- *roots* — anterior primary rami of C5–T1 spinal nerves
- *trunks* — the *upper trunk* formed from roots C5 and C6, the *middle trunk* by C7 and the *lower trunk* by the union of roots C8 and T1
- *divisions* — each trunk separates into *anterior* and *posterior* divisions
- *cords* — the anterior divisions of upper and middle trunks join to form the lateral cord, the anterior division of the lower trunk continues as the medial cord and the posterior divisions of all three trunks join together to form the posterior cord
- *branches* — major branches from each cord have already been identified.

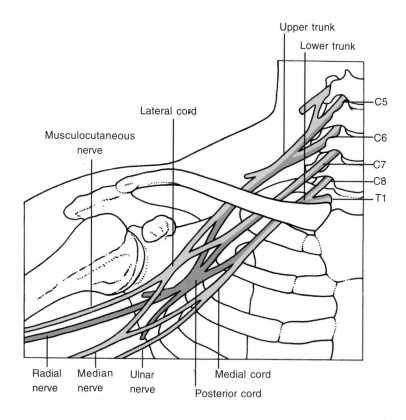

Fig. 5.4 **The brachial plexus.** The anterior division is shown in light orange, the posterior division in dark yellow

Trace each cord of the brachial plexus proximally and note the divisions contributing to their formation. Identify again the trunks of the brachial plexus in the posterior triangle and trace them medially to the roots contributing to their formation (Figs 5.3, 5.4).

Identify the *serratus anterior* muscle on the medial wall of the axilla. By blunt dissection expose the long thoracic nerve on its superficial surface (Fig. 5.1). Trace the nerve towards its origin from the roots as much as possible. Clean the surface of the serratus anterior. Note that the muscle arises by finger-like processes or digitations from the upper eight ribs. Follow the muscle to its insertion onto the costal surface of the medial border of the scapula. Note that most of the muscle is inserted onto the inferior angle of the scapula.

∗ The long thoracic nerve is vulnerable as it lies on the medial wall in surgical dissections of the axilla. This will result in a prominent medial border of the scapula, a condition known as winging of the scapula. The inferior angle will be the most prominent part.

Detachment of the limb

Turn the cadaver over onto its front and examine the serratus anterior from the back. Divide the muscle starting from below leaving part of the muscle and its nerve attached to the trunk. A good view of the contents of the axilla can now be had from behind. Identify the structures. Locate the suprascapular nerve branching from the upper trunk (Fig. 5.2) and trace it to the suprascapular notch on the upper border of the scapula, medial to the coracoid process. The nerve is accompanied by the suprascapular artery which is a branch of the subclavian artery. Divide both the nerve and the suprascapular artery. Divide also the accessory nerve and the accompanying vessels which are under the trapezius muscle. Identify again the levator scapulae and divide the levator scapulae near its insertion to the upper part of the medial border of the scapula. Abduct the arm and divide the latissimus dorsi on the posterior wall of the axilla near the trunk.

Turn the cadaver onto its back. Tie the axillary vessels and the brachial plexus with a piece of string very near the clavicle and divide them. The upper limb can now be detached by dividing the small vessels and folds of skin which attach it to the trunk.

6

The front and back of the arm

Skin reflection

Make a circular incision at the middle of the forearm and connect this by a vertical incision to the cut end of the skin in the middle of the arm. Reflect the skin carefully taking care to preserve the superficial veins.

The cubital fossa

The cubital fossa in front of the elbow is bounded laterally by the *brachioradialis* muscle and medially by the *pronator teres* (Fig. 6.1).

✳ Superficial veins here are often used for intravenous injections. Such injections can inadvertently be made into the brachial artery or the median nerve which are closely related to the veins with disastrous consequences.

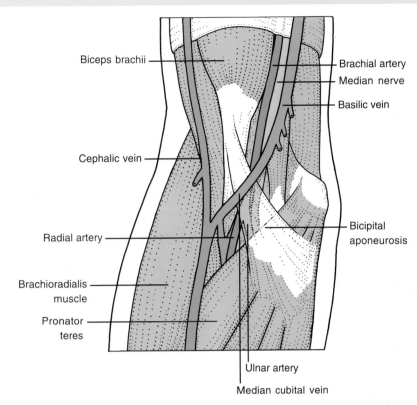

Fig. 6.1 **Structures of the cubital fossa (right side)**

Identify the tendon of biceps in the cubital fossa. Note its flat prolongation onto the deep fascia, the *bicipital aponeurosis* which separates the superficial veins (variable in their patterns) from the brachial artery and the median nerve (Fig. 6.1 and 6.2). Clean the superficial veins, the biceps tendon and its aponeurosis and also the brachial artery and the median nerve in the cubital fossa.

The floor of the cubital fossa is formed by the *brachialis* and the *supinator* muscles and its roof by the deep fascia and the *bicipital aponeurosis*. It contains the *biceps tendon*, the *brachial artery* and its terminal branches (radial and ulnar arteries) and the *median* and the *radial* nerves. A prominent superficial vein, the *median cubital vein*, connecting the *cephalic* and the *basilic* veins lies superficial to the bicipital aponeurosis. Both the cephalic and the basilic veins are the two major superficial veins of the upper limb and they commence as a continuation of the dorsal venous arch at the back of the hand. In the arm the cephalic vein lies along the lateral border of the biceps and the basilic vein along its medial border.

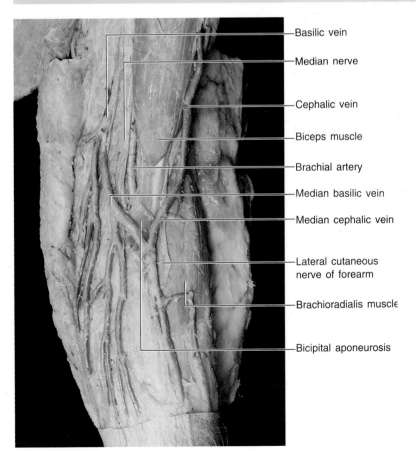

Fig. 6.2 **Dissection of the left cubital fossa**

Surface and living anatomy

Bend your elbow and identify the
tendon of biceps in the cubital fossa.
Now straighten the elbow and feel
the pulsation of the brachial artery
medial to the biceps tendon. The
median nerve lies medial to the
artery.

Remove the deep fascia from the
front of the arm and by blunt dissection separate *biceps brachii,
coracobrachialis* and *brachialis* (Fig.
6.3). The *musculocutaneous nerve*
enters coracobrachialis and is a
guide to its identification. Trace the
nerve into the muscle and clean its
branches. It supplies coracobrachialis, biceps and brachialis and
continues as *lateral cutaneous* nerve
of the forearm (Fig. 6.2). Trace the
median nerve and the brachial artery
downwards. Note that the nerve lies
lateral to the artery in the upper part
of the arm and that it crosses to its
medial side as it descends. Clean the
branches of the artery. *Profunda
brachii* is its biggest branch and it
accompanies the radial nerve.

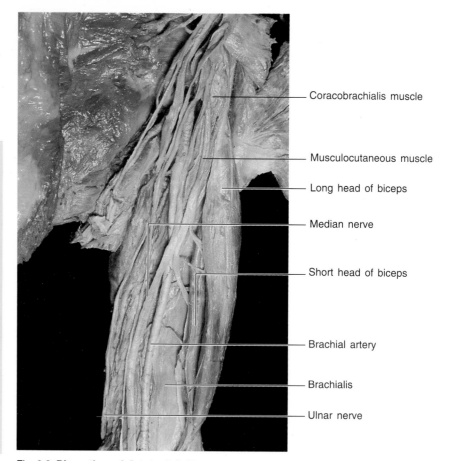

Fig. 6.3 **Dissection of front of (left) arm**

Labels on figure:
- Coracobrachialis muscle
- Musculocutaneous muscle
- Long head of biceps
- Median nerve
- Short head of biceps
- Brachial artery
- Brachialis
- Ulnar nerve

The brachialis muscle lies deep to
biceps. Brachialis takes origin from
the lower half of the front of the
shaft of the humerus and its insertion
is into the coronoid process of the
ulna.

Biceps has two heads of origin, the
long head from the supraglenoid
tubercle of the scapula inside the
capsule of the shoulder joint and the
short head from the coracoid process
of the scapula. It is inserted by a
tendon into the tuberosity of the
radius and also by the bicipital
aponeurosis into the deep fascia of
the forearm.

Brachialis and biceps flex the
elbow joint and the latter is also a
powerful supinator of the forearm.
Attachments of these muscles will be
examined later.

✱ Brachial artery may be
compressed against the humerus
anywhere in the arm to control
bleeding from the forearm and
hand. The best place for this is
the middle of the arm.

✱ Brachial artery is usually used
for measuring the blood pressure.
A stethoscope is kept over the
artery in the cubital fossa after
occluding the artery in the middle
of the arm by inflating the cuff of
the sphygmomanometer.

In the arm the basilic vein, the
brachial artery and the median
nerve lie along the medial border
of the biceps muscle. A careless
incision placed along the medial
border of the muscle may damage
all these structures.

Remove the skin and the deep fascia from the back of the arm and clean the triceps muscle (Fig. 6.4). Identify the long head of triceps. It takes origin from the infraglenoid tubercle of the scapula. The part of the muscle lateral to the long head is the lateral head of the triceps.

Identify the radial nerve in the axilla. Trace the nerve into triceps and note that it disappears under the lateral head. Insert a forceps along the course of the nerve under the lateral head of triceps and cut the muscle over the forceps without damaging the nerve. Reflection of the lower cut portion of the lateral head will reveal the nerve winding round the humerus in its radial groove (Fig. 6.5). The radial nerve may be damaged in fractures of the shaft of the humerus where the nerve lies directly on the bone. Triceps in this case will not be paralysed totally as it receives one or two branches from the radial nerve in the axilla.

Part of the triceps taking origin from the humerus below the radial nerve is the medial head of triceps. Clean the branches of the radial nerve to the three heads of triceps. Also verify the insertion of triceps onto the superior surface of the olecranon process of the ulna.

Finally expose the ulnar nerve behind the medial epicondyle. Trace it upwards to its origin in the brachial plexus. Note that the ulnar and median nerves do not give off branches in the arm.

∗ Three nerves are prone to injury in the arm as they lie closely related to the humerus; the axillary nerve as it winds around the surgical neck, the radial nerve as it lies in the radial (spiral) groove and the ulnar nerve as it lies behind the medial epicondyle.

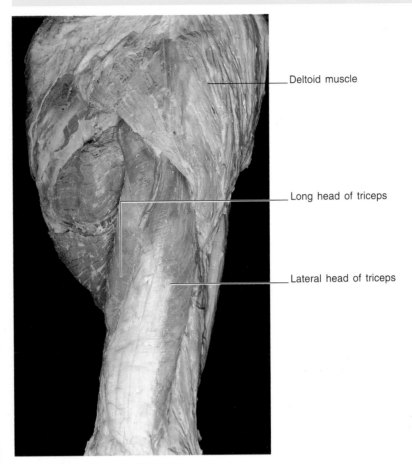

Deltoid muscle

Long head of triceps

Lateral head of triceps

Fig. 6.4 **Back of the arm (left side)**

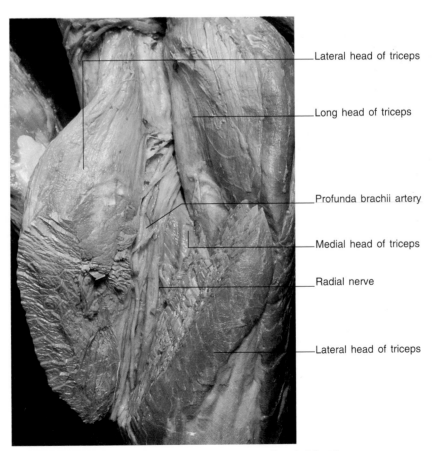

Lateral head of triceps

Long head of triceps

Profunda brachii artery

Medial head of triceps

Radial nerve

Lateral head of triceps

Fig. 6.5 **Back of the left arm after reflection of the lateral head of the triceps**

7

The shoulder region

In this dissection you will study the structures around the shoulder joint and then examine the joint itself. *Deltoid* is the massive muscle covering the shoulder joint and the reflection of it will expose the muscles connecting the scapula to the humerus, viz. *supraspinatus, infraspinatus, subscapularis,* and *teres minor.* Tendons of these muscles fuse with the capsule of the shoulder joint and form the '*rotator cuff*' which stabilises the shoulder joint.

Deltoid muscle

Examine the deltoid muscle (Fig. 7.1). Note that it takes origin from the clavicle, the acromion and the spine of the scapula and that it is inserted onto the deltoid tuberosity at the middle of the humerus. The fibres arising from the acromion have a multi-pennate arrangement making this a powerful muscle.

Reflection of deltoid

Detach deltoid from the clavicle, the acromion and the spine of the scapula and reflect it towards its insertion. Make sure that the axillary nerve supplying the muscle and the posterior circumflex humeral artery accompanying the nerve are not damaged during reflection.

Clean the axillary nerve (p.13) and the posterior circumflex humeral artery. These pass through the *quadrilateral space* before entering the deltoid muscle (Fig. 7.2). By blunt dissection define the boundaries of the quadrilateral space. It is bounded above by the shoulder joint and teres minor, below by teres major, medially by the long head of triceps and laterally by the surgical neck of humerus.

Clean the long head of triceps. Trace it between teres major and teres minor to its origin from the infraglenoid tubercle of the scapula. Similarly clean teres major and trace it to its insertion on the shaft of the humerus.

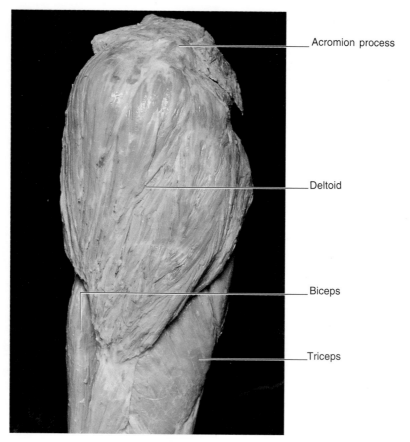

Fig. 7.1 **Lateral aspect of the left shoulder**

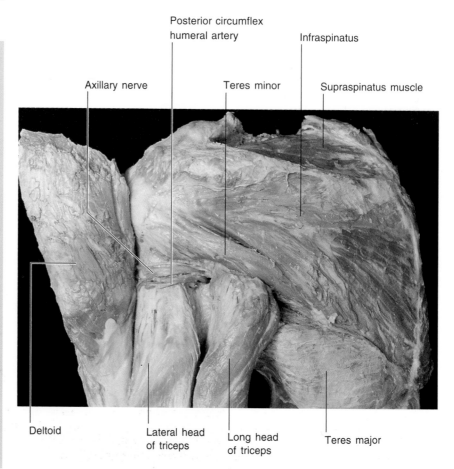

Fig. 7.2 **Structures deep to the deltoid muscle**

Now examine the supraspinatus muscle taking origin from the supraspinous fossa of the scapula. Clean the muscle and note that it goes under the *coraco-acromial ligament* before it is inserted onto the capsule of the shoulder joint and the greater tubercle of the humerus .

✳ Inflammation of the supraspinatus tendon (tendinitis) will cause pain in the middle range of abduction as the swollen tendon impinges against the acromion and the coraco-acromial ligament producing the 'painful arc'. The subacromial bursa separates the tendon of supraspinatus from the coraco-acromial ligament.

Clean the infraspinatus (Fig. 7.2). Identify the suprascapular nerve (p.14) and the accompanying artery. Lift up the upper border of supraspinatus medial to the coracoid process and trace the nerve under the muscle into the supraspinous fossa (Fig. 7.3). The suprascapular nerve supplies supraspinatus. It can then be traced into the infraspinous fossa of the scapula where it supplies the infraspinatus muscle. Infraspinatus takes origin from the infraspinous fossa and is inserted into the posterior surface of the greater tubercle.

Clean teres minor extending from the lateral border of the scapula to its insertion onto the capsule of the shoulder joint and the greater tubercle below the insertion of infraspinatus. It is supplied by the axillary nerve.

Turn the limb over and clean the subscapular muscle on the ventral surface of the scapula. Trace it to its insertion onto the lesser tubercle.

Shoulder joint

Cut through the tendon of subscapularis near its insertion and reflect the muscle medially to expose the anterior aspect of the capsule of the shoulder joint. Note the long head of biceps piercing the capsule (Fig. 7.4). Note that there is no muscle reinforcing the capsule below the subscapularis.

✳ The lower part of the capsule is commonly torn when falling on the outstretched hand producing a dislocation of the shoulder joint. The axillary nerve lying below the joint may be damaged in this injury.

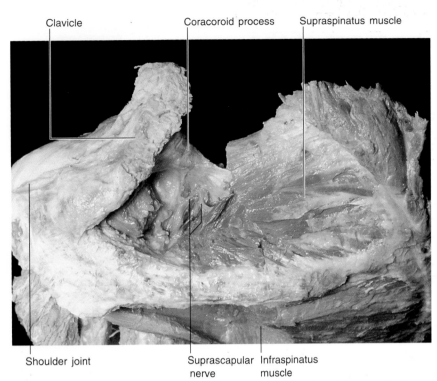

Fig. 7.3 **The left shoulder region after reflection of deltoid and partial removal of the supraspinatus muscle**

Cut through the capsule and laterally rotate the humerus to open the joint. Trace the long head of biceps to its origin from the supraglenoid tubercle of the scapula inside the joint. Notice the glenoid labrum, a fibro cartilage, on the margin of the glenoid.

SURFACE AND LIVING ANATOMY

Examine your partner's shoulder. Note its rounded contour contributed by the deltoid muscle and the upper end of the humerus. Dislocation of the humerus will result in a flattening of the lateral aspect of the shoulder making the acromion very prominent.

Move the arm forwards. This is flexion of the arm at the shoulder joint and the opposite movement is extension. Abduction is the movement when the arm is moved laterally away from the trunk and when it is brought towards the trunk it is known as adduction. The humerus can also be rotated medially and laterally around a vertical axis.

The lesser tubercle rotates inwards in medial rotation and outwards in lateral rotation.

Combinations of the above mentioned movements are possible to perform various functions. When combing your hair the shoulder is abducted and laterally rotated. To scratch the lower part of your back you adduct and medially rotate the shoulder joint.

Finally, note that the wide range of movement at the shoulder requires movement of the scapula and the clavicle. Hold the scapula and prevent it from moving. The shoulder can now be abducted to about 90 degrees only.

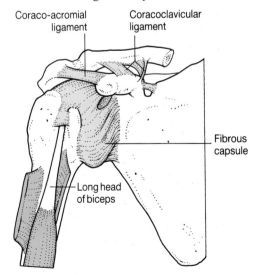

Fig. 7.4 **The right shoulder joint**

8

The front of the forearm

Skin reflection

Make a vertical incision on the remaining skin on the forearm and reflect the skin after a second incision along the distal skin crease of the forearm.

In the superficial fascia the cephalic vein will be exposed. The vein is formed in the dorsal venous arch at the back of the hand and crosses the lateral border of the distal aspect of the forearm lying on the radius (Fig. 8.1) where it has a more or less constant position and can be used for intravenous injections.

Remove the deep fascia and expose the superficial muscles of the front of the forearm. Clean them and identify them by referring to Figures 8.1 and 8.2. Examine the muscles taking origin from the *medial epicondyle* of the humerus (common flexor origin). These are pronator teres, *flexor carpi radialis*, palmaris longus (may not be always present) and the flexor carpi ulnaris. At a slightly deeper plane you will see the *flexor digitorum superficialis*. Insertions of these muscles (Fig. 8.2) can be verified later. Actions of the muscles are implied in their names Flexor carpi radialis and flexor carpi ulnaris flex the carpus or the wrist whereas flexor digitorum superficialis flexes the digits (the fingers).

Clean *brachioradialis* on the lateral aspect of the forearm. It takes origin from the lateral supracondylar ridge of the humerus and is inserted onto the distal end of the radius just above its styloid process. It is a flexor of the elbow and is supplied by the radial nerve.

The superficial muscles should now be reflected to demonstrate the deeper structures.

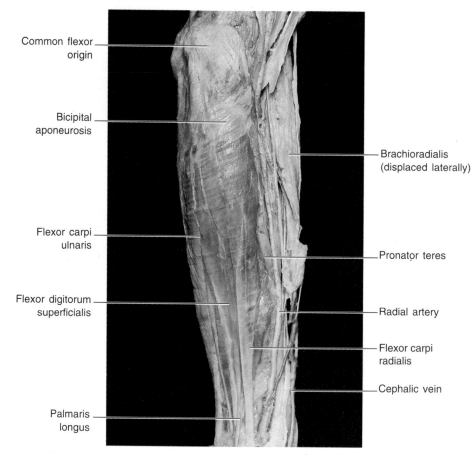

Common flexor origin

Bicipital aponeurosis

Flexor carpi ulnaris

Flexor digitorum superficialis

Palmaris longus

Brachioradialis (displaced laterally)

Pronator teres

Radial artery

Flexor carpi radialis

Cephalic vein

Fig. 8.1 **Superficial structures of the front of forearm (left side)**

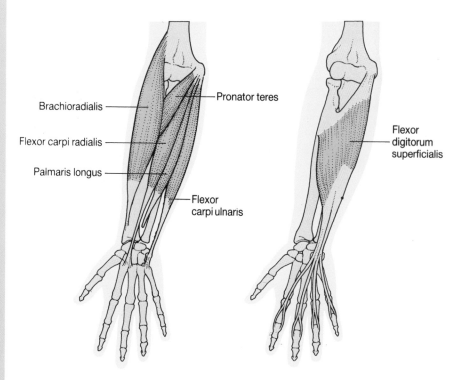

Brachioradialis

Flexor carpi radialis

Palmaris longus

Pronator teres

Flexor carpi ulnaris

Flexor digitorum superficialis

Fig. 8.2 **Flexor muscles of the front of the forearm: superficial layer (right side)**

Cut flexor carpi radialis in its lower third and pronator teres near its insertion to the radius. Push these two muscles medially. Retract brachioradialis and the accompanying extensor carpi radialis longus laterally and expose the radial artery (Fig. 8.3). The brachial artery divides into the radial and ulnar arteries in the cubital fossa. Clean the radial artery and note that it lies lateral to flexor carpi radialis at the wrist where its pulsation is usually felt. Identify the muscles on which the radial artery lies. The artery lies on the muscles attached to the radius. In the upper part of the forearm from above downwards these are *supinator*, *pronator teres* and the radial head of flexor digitorum superficialis (Fig. 8.3).

Identify the radial head of flexor digitorum superficialis and reflect it without damaging the underlying muscle. Do this by inserting a forceps under the muscle to be incised and cutting on to the forceps. The superficial muscles of the forearm can now be pushed to one side or even removed to expose the deep muscles.

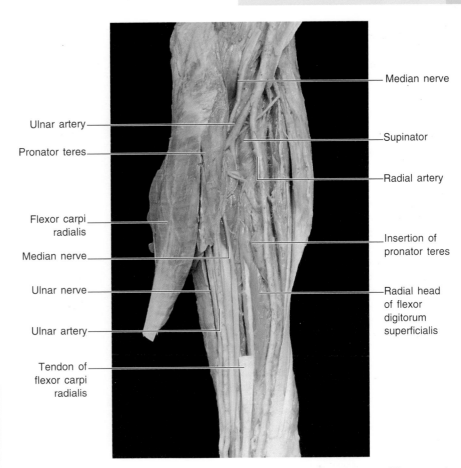

Fig. 8.3 **Structures in front of the forearm after reflection of the pronator teres and flexor carpi radialis (left side)**

There are three deep muscles in the front of the forearm. Identify *flexor pollicis longus* (pollex = thumb) on the lateral aspect and *flexor digitorum profundus* (profundus = deep) medially (Fig. 8.4). Separate these muscles from each other in the distal part of the forearm and expose a transverse running muscle, *pronator quadratus.*

Clean the median nerve from the cubital fossa downwards and note its course and branches. The nerve leaves the cubital fossa by going through pronator teres (between its superficial and deep heads). Note that in the lower part of the forearm it lies medial to flexor carpi radialis, deep to palmaris longus. The nerve can be blocked by local anaesthetics at this position.

The median nerve supplies pronator teres, palmaris longus flexor carpi radialis and flexor digitorum superficialis. Its anterior interosseus branch supplies flexor pollicis longus, the lateral half of flexor digitorum profundus and pronator quadratus.

Separate flexor pollicis longus and flexor digitorum profundus in the upper part of the forearm and expose the interosseus membrane connecting the radius and the ulna. Clean the anterior interosseus nerve accompanied by an artery lying on the membrane. Trace the branches of the nerve to the muscles and also note its origin from the median nerve.

The innervation of the muscles in the front of the forearm can be summarized: all are supplied by the median nerve except flexor carpi ulnaris, the medial half of flexor digitorum profundus and brachioradialis.

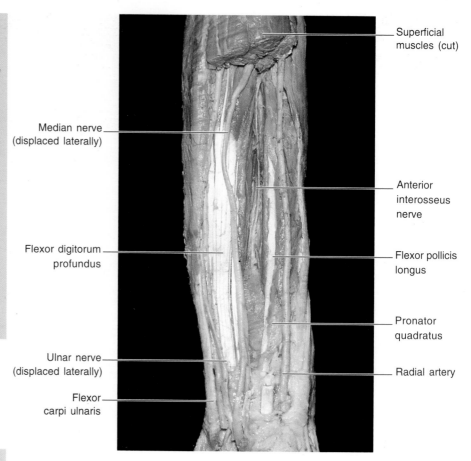

Fig. 8.4 **Deep structures in the front of the forearm (left side)**

Median nerve (displaced laterally)

Flexor digitorum profundus

Ulnar nerve (displaced laterally)

Flexor carpi ulnaris

Superficial muscles (cut)

Anterior interosseus nerve

Flexor pollicis longus

Pronator quadratus

Radial artery

Brachioradialis is supplied by the radial nerve just above the elbow. The ulnar nerve supplies flexor carpi ulnaris and the medial half of profundus.

Clean the ulnar nerve and trace its branches to the flexor carpi ulnaris and flexor digitorum profundus. It lies medial to the ulnar artery (the nerve is displaced laterally in Fig. 8.4 for better exposure). Clean the ulnar artery and note its course.

✳ The ulnar nerve can be damaged at the elbow and at the wrist where it lies superficially.

9

The palm of the hand

OSTEOLOGY

Refer to Figure 9.1 and familiarize yourself with the bones of the hand.

Skin reflection

Incise the skin along the medial and lateral borders of the hand and also make a curved incision along the roots of the fingers. Reflect the skin taking special care not to remove the palmar aponeurosis and the superficial nerves and vessels (Fig. 9.2). Note that the skin of the palm is adherent to the underlying connective tissue. The fixity will prevent the skin from slipping over objects whilst gripping. Remove also the skin from the front of the fingers and thumb preserving the digital nerves and vessels and the fibrous flexor sheath covering the flexor tendons.

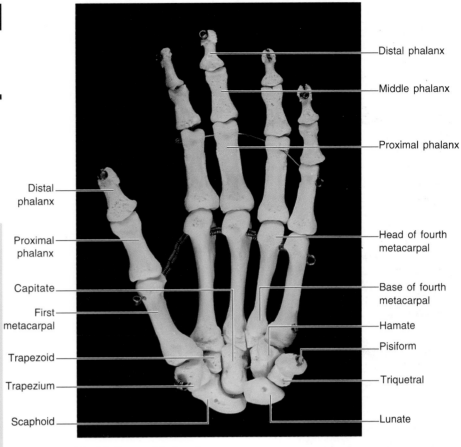

Fig. 9.1 **Bones of the hand**

Palmar aponeurosis (Fig. 9.2)

The palmar aponeurosis lies immediately deep to the skin of the palm. It extends distally from the flexor retinaculum and divides into four slips, one to each finger, to be attached to the flexor sheath.

∗ The palmar aponeurosis is clinically important as it can be affected by Dupuytren's contracture in its medial part. It undergoes fibrosis and will produce flexion deformity of the medial two fingers.

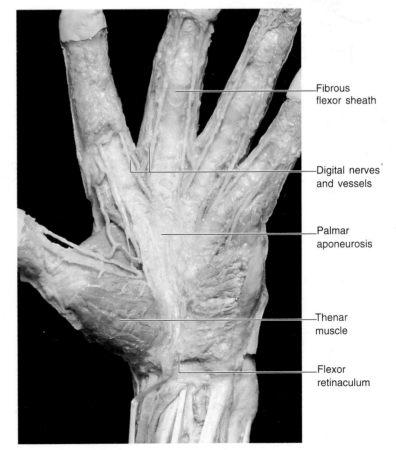

Fig. 9.2 **Superficial structures in the palm**

Carpal tunnel

The carpal tunnel is the space between the flexor retinaculum, a thickening of the deep fascia which prevents 'bow stringing' of the flexor tendons (Figs 9.2, 9.3 & 9.4) and the carpal bones. The space is packed with tendons entering the hand. The median nerve goes through the tunnel.

✳ The median nerve can be compressed by swelling of the tendons or by arthritis affecting the joints of the carpal bones increasing pressure in the tunnel. The condition is known as *carpal tunnel syndrome* which manifests as pain and diminished sensation on the skin along the distribution of the median nerve as well as weakness of the thenar muscles. These muscles are supplied by the median nerve. The ulnar nerve lies superficial to the retinaculum and is not affected in carpal tunnel syndrome.

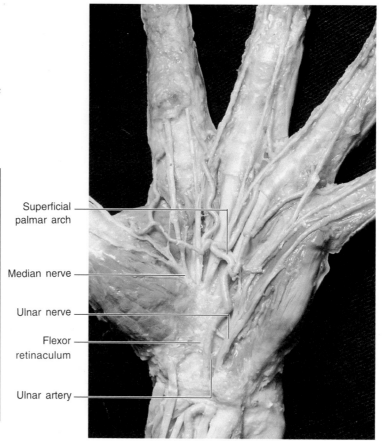

Fig. 9.3 **Superficial palmar arch**

Superficial palmar arch (Fig. 9.3)

Remove the palmar aponeurosis and expose the superficial palmar arch, the arterial arcade formed by the ulnar artery with a small contribution from the radial artery. The digital branches of the ulnar and the median nerves will now also be exposed. Clean them and also the digital branches of the superficial palmar arch.

Median and ulnar nerves (Fig. 9.4)

These two nerves supply the intrinsic muscles and the skin of the palm of the hand. The palmar digital branches at the distal aspect wind round the fingers to supply the skin on the dorsum of the terminal phalanges as well. The skin on the palm of the hand is supplied by palmar cutaneous branches that are given off from the main trunks (median and ulnar) in the forearm. Therefore in injuries of the median or ulnar nerves at the wrist the palmar branches may escape and hence sensation in the palm of the hand may not be affected.

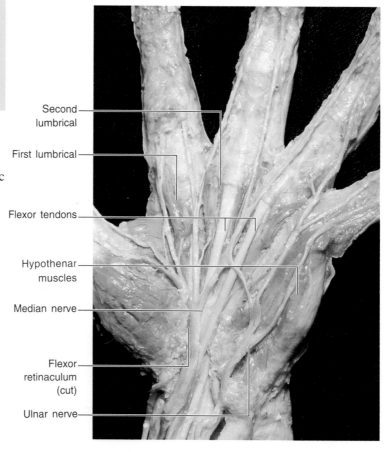

Fig. 9.4 **Median and the ulnar nerves in the hand**

Remove the superficial palmar arch carefully to expose the median and ulnar nerves more fully. Refer to Figure 9.4 and trace the branches of the two nerves. The skin on the lateral three and a half fingers are supplied by the digital branches from the median nerve and the medial one and a half by the ulnar nerve. This distribution however is variable and there may also be connections between the two nerves as seen in Figure 9.4. The muscular branches of the nerves are distributed as follows. The three thenar muscles (see below) and the lateral two lumbrical muscles are supplied by the median nerve. All the other intrinsic muscles of the hand are supplied by the ulnar nerve.

Refer to Figure 9.4 and clean the muscular branches from the median nerve to the thenar muscles and the first two lumbrical muscles. Incise the flexor retinaculum and note the position of the median nerve in the carpal tunnel. Also note that the ulnar nerve with the ulnar artery lying lateral to it crosses superficial to the flexor retinaculum and hence is outside the tunnel.

Thenar muscles (Fig. 9.5)

The thenar muscles are a group of three muscles, viz. the abductor pollicis brevis, the flexor pollicis brevis and opponens.

Verify the insertion of the abductor and the flexor to the lateral aspect of the first phalanx of the thumb. Reflect these two muscles to expose the opponens which is inserted onto the first metacarpal bone. More medially is the adductor pollicis which is inserted onto the medial aspect of the first phalanx of the thumb.

These muscles are important in producing a precision grip or pincer grip as in holding a pen. The thumb is first abducted and then flexed and medially rotated at the carpometacarpal joint to bring it into the 'opposed' position. The adductor pollicis is used to exert pressure on the object. The median nerve supplies the three thenar muscles. Adductor pollicis is supplied by the ulnar nerve. Occasionally flexor pollicis brevis may also be supplied by the ulnar nerve.

The hypothenar muscles (Fig. 9.5)

The hypothenar muscles are almost the mirror images of the thenar muscles and are attached to the little finger. The group consists of abductor digiti minimi, flexor digiti minimi and in a deeper plane opponens digiti minimi. The deep branch of the ulnar nerve passes between the flexor and the abductor and supplies all three muscles.

The lumbrical muscles (Figs 9.4 & 9.5)

There are four lumbrical muscles in the hand, one for each finger. Identify them. Note that each muscle takes origin from the flexor digitorum profundus tendon, crosses the root of the finger laterally and is inserted into the dorsal digital expansion at the back of the finger. How the lumbrical muscles of the hand function is not clearly understood. Many are of the view that the muscles are used to simultaneously flex the metacarpophalangeal and extend the interphalangeal joints as in making an upstroke while writing. The lateral two lumbricals are usually supplied by the median nerve and the medial two by the ulnar.

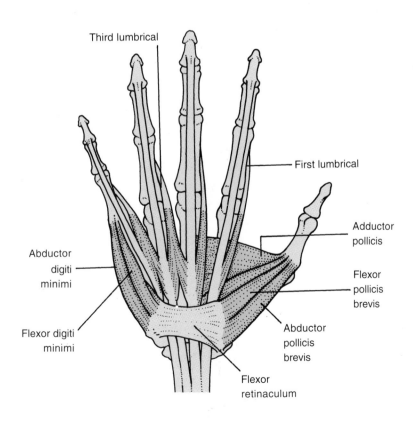

Fig. 9.5 **Thenar and hypothenar muscles, and the lumbricals (right side)**

Insertions of the flexor tendons
(Fig. 9.6)

Trace the tendons of flexor digitorum superficialis and those of the profundus to at least one of the fingers and note their insertions. Verify that at the proximal part of each finger the superficialis is tunnelled through by the profundus tendon. The superficialis is inserted into the base of the middle phalanx and the profundus to the terminal phalanx. Verify the insertions. Also trace the tendon of the flexor pollicis longus to its insertion into the base of the terminal phalanx of the thumb.

The flexor tendons are enclosed by synovial sheaths. The arrangement of these synovial sheaths is illustrated in Figure 9.7.

∗ Synovial sheaths can be infected producing tenosynovitis. Infection can spread throughout the sheath. Infection of the sheath of the little finger can thus spread up to the distal aspect of the forearm.

The flexor tendons are held on to the front of the finger by the fibrous flexor sheath.

∗ The tendons move inside the sheath during flexion and extension. However narrowing of the space in the sheath can occur by thickening of the sheath or nodular thickening of the tendon. The finger may then click painfully when the patient bends it, or when the hand is unclenched the affected finger may remain bent and may suddenly straighten with a snap — 'trigger finger'.

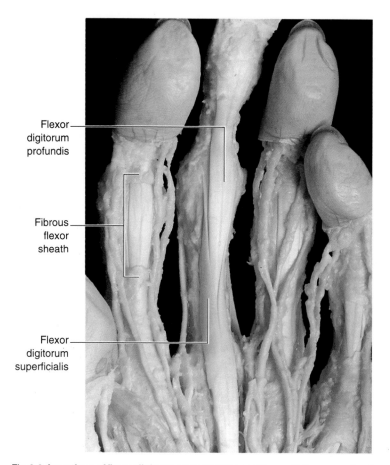

Flexor digitorum profundis

Fibrous flexor sheath

Flexor digitorum superficialis

Fig. 9.6 **Insertions of flexor digitorum superficialis and flexor digitorum profundus**

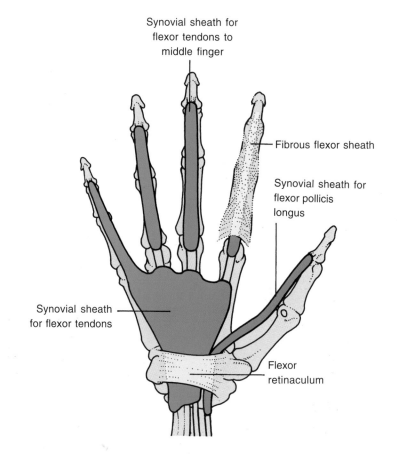

Synovial sheath for flexor tendons to middle finger

Fibrous flexor sheath

Synovial sheath for flexor pollicis longus

Synovial sheath for flexor tendons

Flexor retinaculum

Fig. 9.7 **Arrangement of synovial sheaths for the flexor tendons (right side)**

Deeper aspect of the palm

Cut the flexor tendons at the wrist and reflect them forward (Fig. 9.8) to expose the underlying structures. Clean adductor pollicis, the interossei muscles, the deep palmar arch and the deep branch of the ulnar nerve. Adductor pollicis has a transverse and an oblique head of origin. It is supplied by the deep branch of the ulnar nerve. The deep palmar arch is formed by the radial artery reaching the palm by piercing the first dorsal interosseus muscle in the first interosseus space. The radial artery anastomoses with the deep branch of the ulnar artery to form the deep palmar arch which is smaller than the superficial arch. The interossei muscles lie in the interosseus spaces between the metacarpal bones. Their arrangements are shown in Figure 9.9. The palmar interossei are arranged in such a way that they produce adduction of the fingers by moving them towards the middle finger. The dorsal interossei are abductors of the fingers, i.e. moving the fingers away from the axis of the movement going through the middle of the middle finger. When the palmar and the dorsal interossei act together they, like the lumbricals, can flex the metacarpophalangeal joints and extend the interphalangeal joints. All the interossei are supplied by the deep branch of the ulnar nerve.

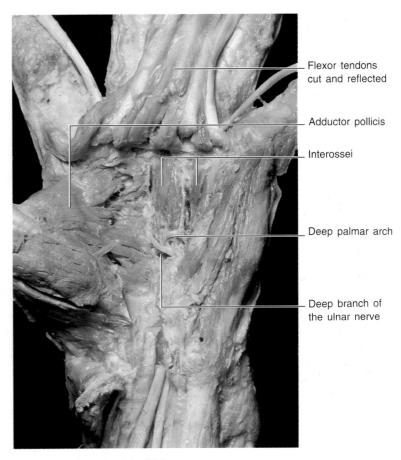

Flexor tendons cut and reflected

Adductor pollicis

Interossei

Deep palmar arch

Deep branch of the ulnar nerve

Fig. 9.8 **Deep structures in the palm (left side)**

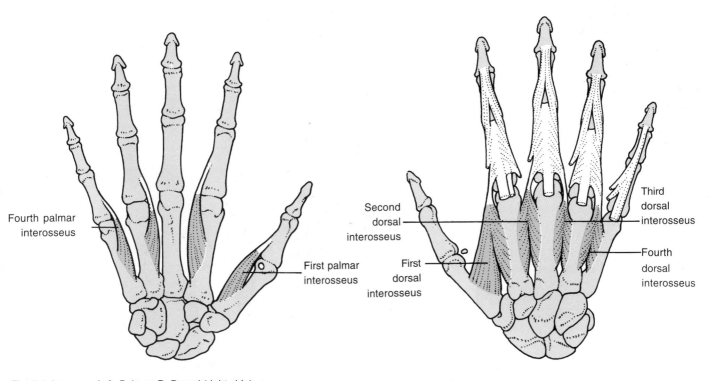

Fourth palmar interosseus

First palmar interosseus

Second dorsal interosseus

First dorsal interosseus

Third dorsal interosseus

Fourth dorsal interosseus

Fig. 9.9 **Interossei. A.** Palmar. **B.** Dorsal (right side)

10

The back of the forearm and dorsum of the hand

Skin reflection

Remove the skin and superficial fascia from the back of the forearm and the hand. Clean the superficial muscles preserving the extensor retinaculum.

The superficial extensor muscles at the back of the forearm are shown in Figure 10.1. Identify the superficial muscles and verify their attachments. *Extensor carpi radialis longus* takes origin from the lateral supracondylar ridge just below the origin of brachioradialis. *Extensor carpi radialis brevis, extensor digitorum, extensor carpi ulnaris* and *extensor digiti minimi* have a common origin from the lateral epicondyle (*common extensor origin*). The extensors of the carpus are inserted into the metacarpal bones; the radial (lateral) extensors into the bases of the first and second metacarpal bones and the ulnar extensor into the fifth metacarpal bone. Extensor digitorum forms the *extensor expansion* at the back of the fingers (see below) and digiti minimi reinforces the extensor expansion at the back of the little finger. All these muscles are supplied by the *posterior interosseus* branch of the *radial nerve*, except extensor carpi radialis longus, which like the brachioradialis is supplied by the radial nerve just above the elbow.

Wrist drop

✳ *Paralysis of the radial nerve* above the elbow will paralyse all the extensors of the wrist. The flexors of the wrist will overact and the wrist will adopt a flexed position, a condition known as *wrist drop*. Note that gripping with the hand is impossible in the flexed position of the wrist.

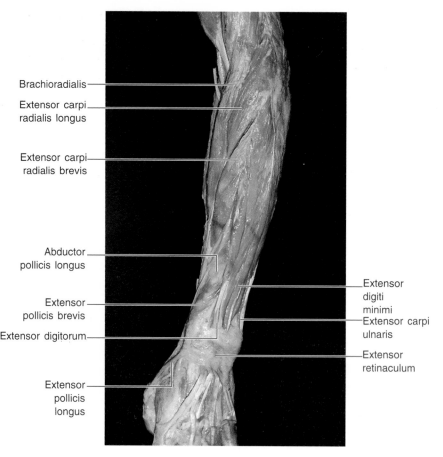

Fig. 10.1 **Superficial muscles of the back of the forearm**

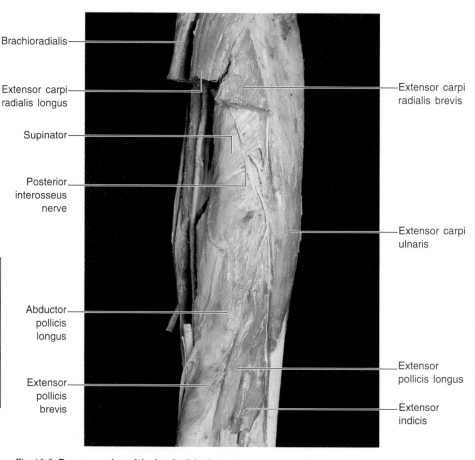

Fig. 10.2 **Deep muscles of the back of the forearm**

The deep extensors

The deep extensor group contains the long abductor and the extensors of the thumb as well as extensor indicis. *Abductor pollicis longus* and *extensor pollicis brevis* can be seen superficially in the distal part of the forearm winding round the radius (Fig. 10.1). Their origins lie deep.

Remove brachioradialis and the superficial extensors and expose supinator. Trace the *posterior interosseus branch of the radial nerve* going through *supinator* and note its branches to the extensor muscles in the forearm (Fig. 10.2). Supinator is inserted into the posterolateral aspect of the upper part of the radius and it supinates the forearm in the extended position.

Clean abductor pollicis longus and extensor pollicis brevis and trace them to their insertions into the bases of the first metacarpal bone and the proximal phalanx of the thumb respectively (Fig. 10.3). Identify *extensor pollicis longus*. Trace its tendon through the extensor retinaculum and note that the tendon winds round medial to the dorsal tubercle of the radius and turns laterally to reach its insertion into the distal phalanx of the thumb.

✳ The tendon of extensor pollicis longus can rupture spontaneously or as a consequence of fracture of the lower end of the radius (*Colles' fracture*). Flexor pollicis longus will then overact producing a flexion deformity of the distal phalanx of the thumb (hammer thumb).

Extensor indicis is an additional extensor for the index finger. Its tendon joins the ulnar side of the extensor digitorum tendon on the index finger. This muscle can be connected to the tendon of extensor pollicis longus to repair a hammer thumb.

Anatomical snuff box (Fig. 10.3)

The space proximal to the thumb bounded medially by extensor pollicis longus and laterally by the tendons of abductor pollicis longus and extensor pollicis brevis is the anatomical snuff box. Extend your thumb and identify the anatomical snuff box. The *scaphoid bone* forms its floor. The *radial artery* lies within it and the cephalic vein crosses it superficially.

Radial artery

Trace the radial artery from the distal aspect of the front of forearm.

It goes deep to the tendons of abductor pollicis and extensor pollicis brevis, lies in the anatomical snuff box and reaches the first interosseus space after crossing deep to the tendon of extensor pollicis longus (Fig. 10.3). The artery then passes between the two heads of the first dorsal interosseus muscle to reach the palm of the hand where it contributes to the formation of the *deep palmar arch*.

✳ After a fall on the outstretched hand, tenderness in the anatomical snuff box is suggestive of a fracture of the scaphoid bone. Scaphoid fractures through its waist (middle portion). The artery to the bone usually enters its distal half and hence when it fractures the proximal half will be without blood supply and may undergo *avascular necrosis*.

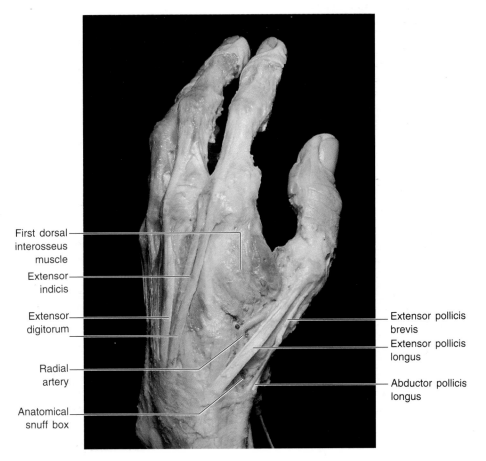

First dorsal interosseus muscle

Extensor indicis

Extensor digitorum

Radial artery

Anatomical snuff box

Extensor pollicis brevis

Extensor pollicis longus

Abductor pollicis longus

Fig. 10.3 **Back of the hand**

Extensor expansion

At the wrist *extensor digitorum* gives
rise to four tendons which supply
digits 2–5. Each slip forms an
expanded hood over the dorsum of
the digit (Fig. 10.4). The expansion
is attached to the base of the
proximal phalanx before dividing
into a *central* and *two marginal slips*.
The central slip is inserted into the
base of the middle phalanx. The
marginal slips unite together and
insert onto the base of the distal
phalanx. The *interossei* and the
lumbricals are inserted into the
proximal part of the extensor
expansion. Verify these attachments.

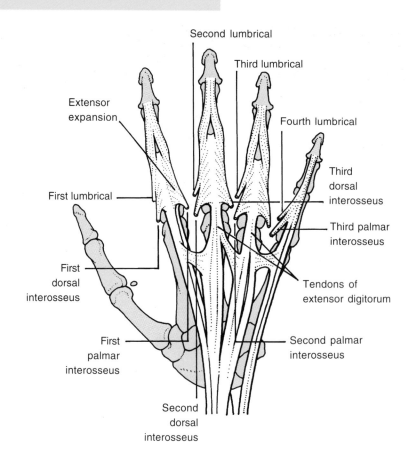

Fig. 10.4 **Extensor tendons of the digits (right side)**

11

The joints of the forearm and hand

The elbow and the superior radio-ulnar joints

Flexion and extension movements of the forearm take place at the elbow joint. *Brachialis*, *biceps* and *brachioradialis* are the main flexors. *Triceps* extends the joint. At the *superior* and *inferior radio-ulnar joints* the *radius* rotates inwards to produce *pronation* (pronation makes the palm of the hand face backwards in the anatomical position.) This is produced by *pronator teres* and *pronator quadratus*. The opposite movement is *supination* in which the radius rotates outwards. In the flexed position of the elbow, biceps acts as a powerful supinator. Supination is weak when the elbow is extended and is done by the supinator muscle.

OSTEOLOGY

Refer to Figure 11.1 and identify the following in the region of the elbow:

- medial and lateral epicondyles of the humerus
- capitulum and trochlea of the humerus
- head and neck of the radius and the tuberosity of the radius
- coronoid and olecranon processes of the ulna
- trochlear notch on the ulna and the radial and coronoid fossae of the humerus. The olecranon fossa at the back of the humerus.

In the elbow joint, the upper surface of the head of radius articulates with the capitulum of the humerus, and the trochlea of the humerus fits into the trochlear notch of the ulna.

The dissection to expose the capsule of the joint will involve removal of the structures closely related to the joint.

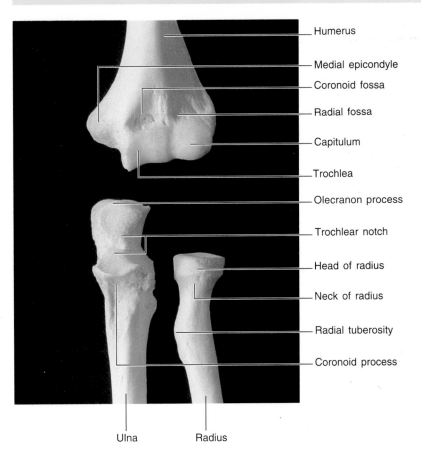

Fig. 11.1 **Lower end of the humerus and the upper ends of the radius and ulna (left side)**

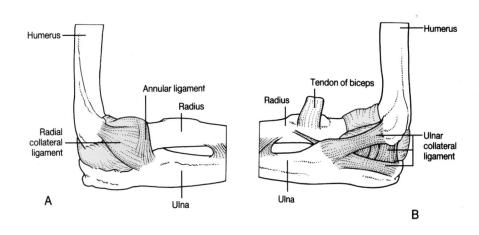

Fig. 11.2 **Right elbow joint. A.** Lateral view. **B.** Medial view

Identify the remains of the brachial artery, the veins, the median and the radial nerves in front of the elbow and remove them. Also verify the insertions of the tendon of biceps to the radial tuberosity and that of the brachialis to the coronoid process. Remove these and expose the front of the capsule of the elbow joint. Similarly expose the rest of the capsule by removing the common flexor origin from the medial epicondyle and the common extensor origin from the lateral epicondyle. Also detach the insertion of triceps from the olecranon. Note that the *ulnar nerve* is lying on the back of the medial epicondyle and the medial collateral ligament and may be damaged in a *posterior dislocation* of the elbow joint. Clean the capsule and define the medial and lateral collateral ligaments (Fig. 11.2). Note that the lateral part of the capsule and the lateral collateral ligaments are attached to the annular ligament and not to the head of the radius.

The upper end of the radius is totally free of ligamentous attachments enabling the radius to rotate freely inside the annular ligament.

Make an incision in front of the capsule and open the joint. Examine the articular surfaces of the humerus, radius and ulna.

In the superior radio-ulnar joint, which shares the capsule of the elbow joint, the head of the radius articulates with the radial notch of the ulna. The two bones are held together by the annular ligament.

Define the annular ligament and note its attachments to the radius. It circles round the head and neck of the radius.

✳ In a young child a sudden pull on the forearm may result in the head of the radius being pulled partly outside the annular ligament. This injury is termed a 'pulled elbow'. In children the head of the radius is not fully formed and the annular ligament is circular. The annular ligament is of conical shape in the adult facilitating a better grip on the radius.

Wrist joint

Refer to Figure 11.3 and identify the bones in the distal part of the forearm and hand.

At the wrist joint the scaphoid, lunate and triquetral bones articulate proximally with the distal end of the radius and the triangular fibrocartilage connecting the distal end of the radius and the ulna. The triangular fibrocartilage separates the wrist joint from the inferior radioulnar joint.

Identify again the structures crossing the wrist in front and at the back. Remove these structures and clean the ligaments and capsule of the joint (Fig. 11.4). Open the capsule and examine the interior of the joint. Note the attachments of the fibrocartilage inside the joint connecting the distal ends of the radius and the ulna.

✳ A fall on the hand may *dislocate the lunate bone* or may dislocate the whole carpus backwards with the lunate remaining stationary (*perilunar dislocation*). These injuries tear the soft tissue and produce avascular necrosis of the bone and may also damage the median nerve.

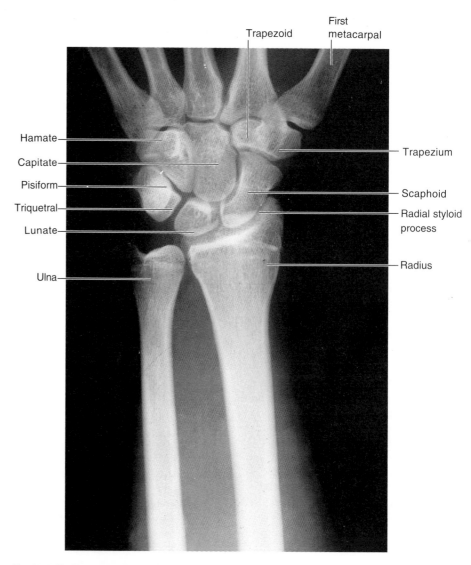

Fig. 11.3 **Radiograph of the wrist in the anatomical position (right side)**

Joints of the hand

Remove the tendons and muscles of the thumb after identifying each of them. Expose the joint between the trapezium and the first metacarpal bone. This is where most of the movements of the thumb takes place. Open the joint and examine the saddle-shaped articular surface of the trapezium.

✻ *Bennett's fracture* is a fracture of the base of the first metacarpal bone involving the carpo-metacarpal joint of the thumb. This is usually sustained as a result of a blow to the point of the thumb as in boxing.

Finally examine the metacarpophalangeal joint and the interphalangeal joints of the thumb and one of the fingers.

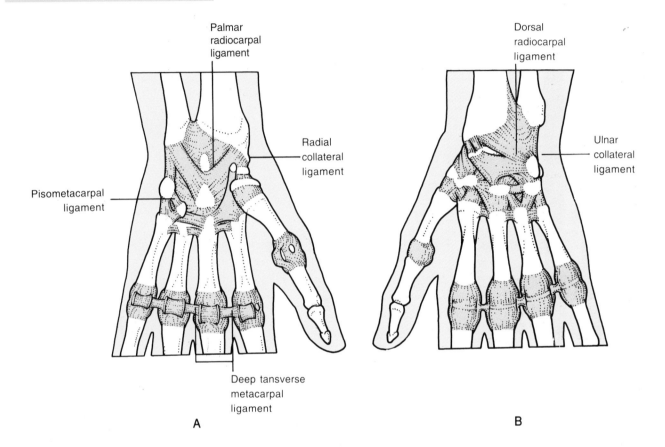

Palmar radiocarpal ligament

Dorsal radiocarpal ligament

Radial collateral ligament

Ulnar collateral ligament

Pisometacarpal ligament

Deep tansverse metacarpal ligament

A

B

Fig. 11.4 **Wrist joint and metacarpals. A.** Anterior view. **B.** Posterior view

THE
THORAX

12

The thoracic cage and intercostal space

In this session we will examine the formation of the thoracic cage, identify important landmarks on the chest wall and also study the anatomy of the intercostal space.

OSTEOLOGY OF THE THORACIC CAGE (Fig. 12.1)

The bony thoracic cage is formed by the 12 thoracic vertebrae at the back, the sternum in front and 12 pairs of ribs in between. The upper 7 pairs of ribs anteriorly articulate directly with the sternum through their respective costal cartilages. The costal cartilages of ribs 8, 9 and 10 articulate with that of the rib above. These ribs with the xiphisternum form the lower costal margin. The *lower most point* of the thoracic cage is the *10th costal cartilage*.

The space between two adjacent ribs is known as the *intercostal space*. Thus there are 11 intercostal spaces on each side.

The junction between the manubrium and the body of the sternum is the *sternal angle*. The second costal cartilage articulates at the sternal angle. The 7th costal cartilage articulates at the junction between the body and the xiphisternum.

Refer to Figure 12.1 and define on an articulated skeleton the components of the bony thoracic cage. Identify the following:

- suprasternal notch
- the sternal angle
- the second costal cartilage
- the lower costal margin.

SURFACE ANATOMY

The sternal angle is palpable on the surface as a transverse ridge (Fig. 12.2). This landmark is used to palpate the second costal cartilage and the second rib. It is possible to identify the other ribs as well as intercostal spaces by counting down from the second rib

Palpate the sternal angle. Identify the costal cartilage, the ribs and

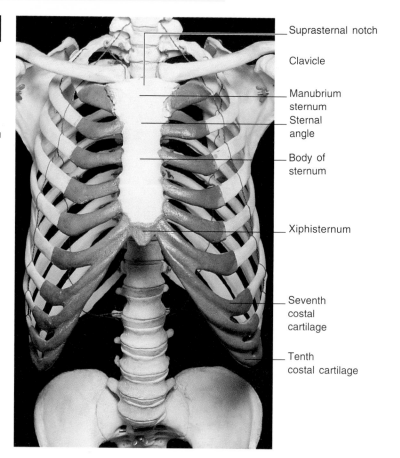

Suprasternal notch

Clavicle

Manubrium sternum

Sternal angle

Body of sternum

Xiphisternum

Seventh costal cartilage

Tenth costal cartilage

Fig. 12.1 **Bony thoracic cage**

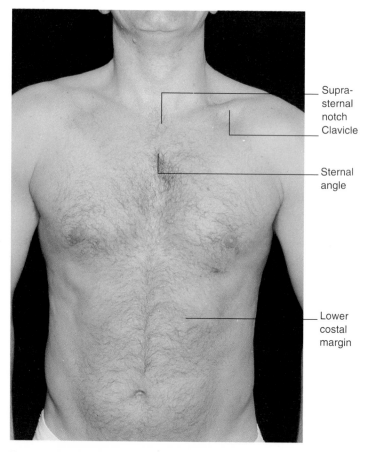

Supra-sternal notch

Clavicle

Sternal angle

Lower costal margin

Fig. 12.2 **Surface anatomy of the chest wall**

intercostal spaces. Note that the first rib is not palpable as it is under the clavicle. Ribs 11 and 12 are rudimentary, confined to the back and are covered by muscles and hence are also not palpable.

Intercostal space

The intercostal space contains the external intercostal, the internal intercostal and the innermost intercostal muscles arranged in three layers. The neurovascular bundle, consisting of the *intercostal nerve* and *vessels*, lies in between the *internal* and the *innermost intercostals*.

Remove the remains of the pectoral muscles and the serratus anterior. Clean the external intercostal muscles in one or two intercostal spaces. Note that the fibres are directed downwards and medially (Figs 12.3 & 12.4). In the anterior part the muscle fibres are replaced by a membrane. Remove the external intercostal muscle exposing the internal intercostal, the fibres of which lie in the opposite direction to those of the external. Remove the internal intercostal muscle and dissect beneath the rib margin to expose the intercostal nerve and vessels. Note the relation of the vein, artery and nerve (Fig. 12.4). The order from above downwards is vein, artery and nerve. All three are protected by the downward projection of the lower border of the rib forming the costal groove.

✳ In cases where it is necessary to insert a chest drain or a needle into the intercostal space it is always placed in the lower part of the space to avoid damage to the neurovascular bundle (which lies along the lower border of the rib along the upper part of the space).

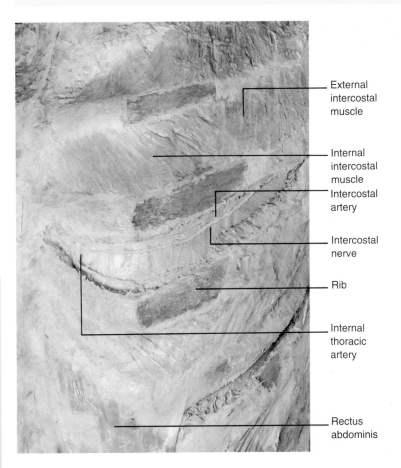

Fig. 12.3 **Intercostal spaces (left side)**

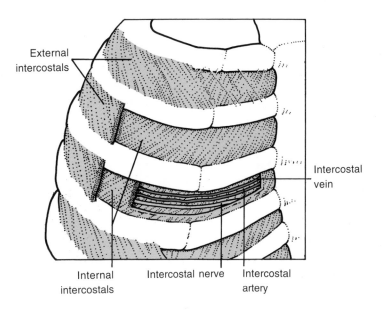

Fig. 12.4 **Intercostal spaces (right side): external view.** The muscles have been partially removed to show the deeper structures

The intercostal nerves are the *anterior rami of the first eleven thoracic nerves*. The course and branches of a typical intercostal nerve is shown in Figure 12.5.

The source and anastomoses of the anterior and posterior intercostal arteries is shown in Figures 12.6 and 12.7. The anterior intercostal arteries are branches of the *internal thoracic artery* or those of its *musculophrenic* branch (Figs 12.3 & 12.7). Most of the posterior intercostal arteries are derived from the descending thoracic aorta.

⁎ Anastomoses between the anterior and posterior intercostal arteries are important collateral channels for circulation in cases of obstruction to the blood flow in the aorta anywhere beyond the origin of the left subclavian artery.

⁎ Coarctation of the aorta is a congenital malformation in which the aorta is constricted. The usual site is in the region of the origin of the left subclavian artery. In coarctation, the intercostal arteries enlarge to facilitate blood flow to the lower part of the body beyond the obstruction. Notching of the ribs is an important radiological sign caused by erosion of the ribs by the dilated intercostal arteries.

Using a bone saw make two transverse cuts on the sternum, one just above the sternal angle and the second at the level of the 5th costal cartilage. Using bone forceps cut ribs 2–6 as posteriorly as possible and also incise the intercostal muscles in between. Cut through the costal cartilages forming the lower costal margin . Detach the deep surface of the sternum and ribs from the underlying fascia and pleura and remove the anterior part of the rib cage in one piece. You may have to incise the muscles in the first intercostal space to do this.

On the inside of the detached part, expose the internal thoracic artery and its branches as well as the accompanying veins (Fig. 12.7).

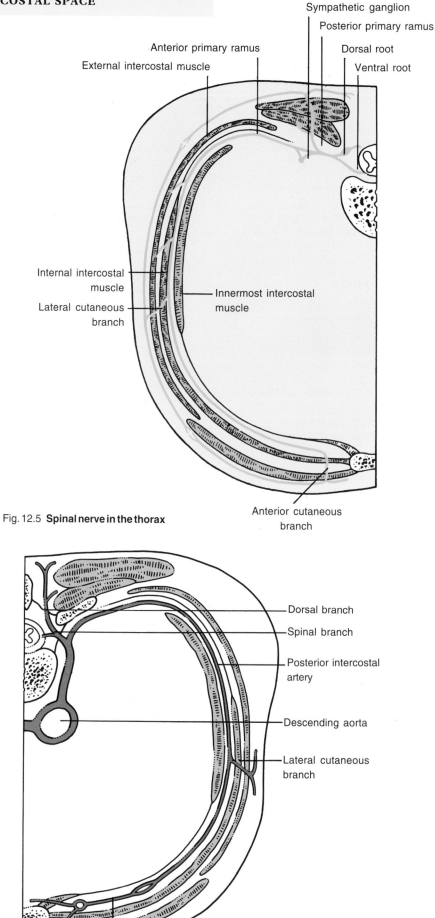

Fig. 12.5 **Spinal nerve in the thorax**

Fig. 12.6 **Arteries in the intercostal space**

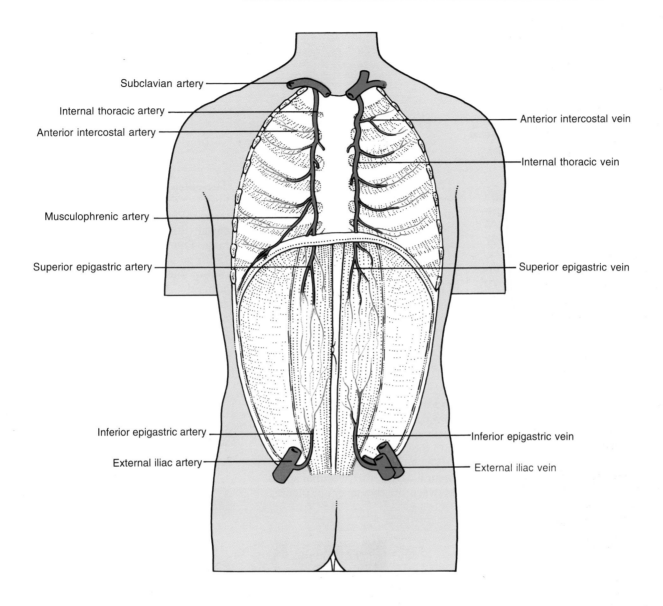

Subclavian artery

Internal thoracic artery

Anterior intercostal artery

Musculophrenic artery

Superior epigastric artery

Inferior epigastric artery

External iliac artery

Anterior intercostal vein

Internal thoracic vein

Superior epigastric vein

Inferior epigastric vein

External iliac vein

Fig. 12.7 **Internal thoracic artery and vein and the anastomoses in the rectus sheath**

13

The thoracic cavity, lungs and pleura

The thoracic cavity contains on either side the right and left lungs surrounded by the pleural cavities and the *mediastinum* in between. We will examine the lungs and pleural cavities in this session and the mediastinum in the subsequent ones.

Lungs and pleural cavities

The right lung is subdivided into three lobes and the left lung into two. The left lung is divided into upper and lower lobes by the oblique fissure. The right lung has an oblique fissure and a horizontal fissure dividing it into upper, middle and lower lobes. Each lung has an apex which extends about 3 cm above the clavicle into the neck, a costal surface, a mediastinal surface and a base or diaphragmatic surface.

The anterior border of the lung separates the costal and the mediastinal surfaces whereas the lower border is between the costal and the diaphragmatic surface.

Each lung is connected to the mediastinum by the root of the lung. The root of the lung contains the main bronchus branching off from the trachea, one pulmonary artery, two pulmonary veins, bronchial arteries supplying the bronchus, and lymph nodes draining the lung.

The right bronchus is shorter, wider and more vertical than the left and therefore foreign bodies getting into the trachea tend to go more easily into the right bronchus than into the left.

The lung is surrounded by the pleural cavity, the potential space between the two layers of pleura.

The outer *parietal* layer of pleura lines the thoracic cavity and the inner *visceral* or *pulmonary* layer closely fits on to the surface of the lung. The two layers become continuous with each other at the root of the lung. The parietal pleura lining the diaphragm is known as the *diaphragmatic pleura* and that lining the mediastinum as the *mediastinal pleura*.

Identify the mediastinum, lungs and the pleura. Define the parietal and the visceral layers of pleura and the pleural cavity which is now opened up. Pull the lung laterally and identify the *root of the lung* (Fig. 13.1).

Define the borders and surfaces of the right and left lung. Replace the thoracic cage and note the extent of the various borders.

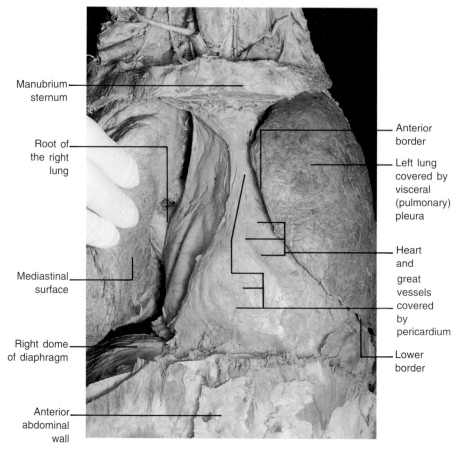

Fig. 13.1 **Lungs and mediastinum**

SURFACE ANATOMY (Fig. 13.2)

Define the borders of the right and left lung and the pleural cavities on your partner.

The apex of the lung and the surrounding pleural cavity extends about 3 cm above the medial part of the clavicle. The apical pleura is covered by a fascia, the *suprapleural membrane* (Sibson's fascia) which is attached to the inner border of the first rib. This fascia prevents the lung and pleura expanding too much into the neck during deep inspiration.

From the apex, the anterior border of the pleural cavity descends behind the sternoclavicular joint to reach the midline at the level of the sternal angle.(Here the two pleural cavities are close to each other.) The anterior limit of the right pleural cavity descends vertically downwards in the midline from the sternal angle to the level of the sixth costal cartilage. From there the lower border extends laterally, crossing the 8th rib in the midclavicular line, 10th rib in the midaxillary line (Fig. 13.2) and then

ascends to the middle of the 12th rib at the back . The posterior border then ascends almost vertically upwards in the paravertebral region.

From the sternal angle the anterior border of the left pleural cavity deviates laterally to the lateral border of the sternum. The extent of the lower and the posterior margins are similar to those on the right.

Surface marking of the lung. The marking of the lung is the same as that of the pleura except for the lower margin and the cardiac notch. The lower margin of the lung is about two ribs higher than the lower margin of the pleura. Because of the bulge of the heart and pericardium, the anterior border of the left lung deviates laterally from the sternal angle to the apex of the heart (usually in the 5th intercostal space, a little inside the midclavicular line) producing the cardiac notch. The oblique fissure lies along the 6th rib and the horizontal fissure on the right side extends from the midaxillary line along the 4th rib.

✳ Knowledge of the extent of the lung and pleura is clinically important. Their lower parts overlap abdominal organs such as the liver, kidney and spleen. On the apical pleura lie the subclavian vessels and the brachial plexus. Procedures such as exposure of the kidney, liver biopsy and canulation of the subclavian vein may inadvertently produce a *pneumothorax* (air in the pleural cavity) resulting in collapse of the lung.

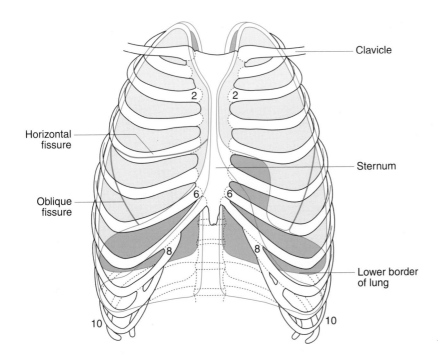

Fig. 13.2 **Surface relationship of the lungs and pleural cavities.** The numbers indicate those of the ribs and costal cartilages

Pull the lung laterally and define the structures at the root of the lung. The root of the lung consists mainly of *two pulmonary veins*, the *pulmonary artery* and the *bronchus* in that order from before backwards. Note that the right main bronchus gives off the *superior lobar bronchus* outside the lung. All the branches of the left bronchus are given off inside the lung.

Incise the structures at the root of the lung. Detach the adhesions between the two layers of pleura and remove the lung. Do this on both sides. Identify the cut ends of the structures at the hilum of the lung (Fig. 13.3) and note their relative positions.

Examine the fissures and lobes of the lung. Replace the lung in the chest cavity and note that the upper lobes (and the middle lobe on the right) face the anterior chest wall whereas the lower lobes are posterior, points worth remembering in examination of the lungs in the living.

Dissect out the main bronchus in the hilum of the lung by removing the lung tissue. Trace the bronchus and clean its branches. Compare the branching pattern to that seen in Figure 13.4.

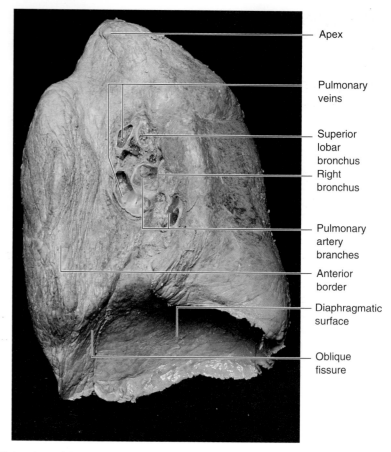

Fig. 13.3 **Medial surface of the right lung**

Each main bronchus gives rise to lobar bronchi that supply the lobes of the lung. Each lobar bronchus gives rise to further branches, segmental bronchi, which ventilate the bronchopulmonary segments. There are ten bronchopulmonary segments in each lung. Each segment has its own branch of the bronchus and pulmonary artery. However, branches of the pulmonary veins and bronchial arteries are intersegmental.

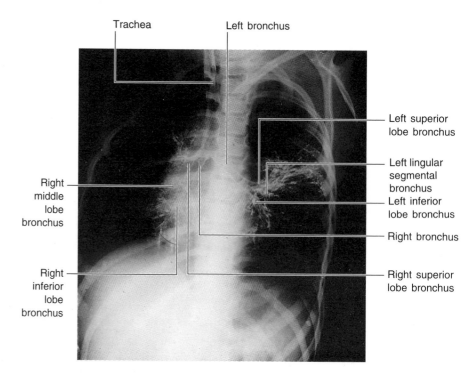

Fig. 13.4 **Bronchogram** (slightly oblique view)

14
The mediastinum

The mediastinum is the region between the two pleural cavities. It contains the heart, great vessels, trachea, oesophagus and many other structures. The mediastinum is divided into four parts for descriptive purposes (Fig. 14.1). The superior mediastinum lies above an imaginary line joining the sternal angle to the lower border of T4. The middle mediastinum contains the heart and pericardium.

The mediastinum is asymmetrical. We will first expose as many of the mediastinal structures as possible on the right and left side. The heart and pericardium and some of the deeply lying structures in the posterior and superior mediastinum will be studied in later dissections.

Refer to Figures 14.2 and 14.3 and expose as many of the structures as possible on the right side. This can be done by carefully peeling away the parietal pleura (mediastinal pleura) still covering these structures.

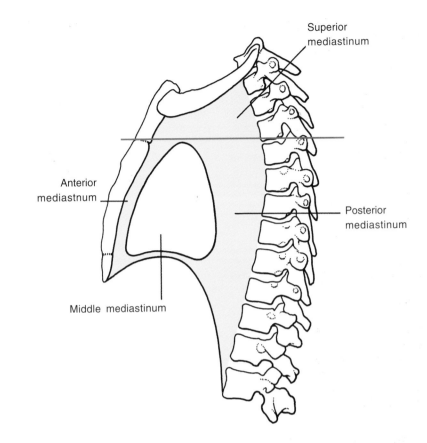

Fig. 14.1 **Divisions of the mediastinum**

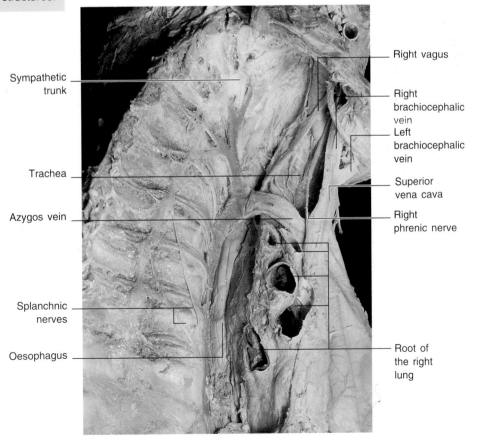

Fig. 14.2 **Right side of the mediastinum**

Brachiocephalic vein and the superior vena cava

The brachiocephalic vein, one on each side, is formed by the union of the *subclavian* and the *internal jugular veins*. The right and left brachiocephalic veins join together to form the *superior vena cava* which drains into the right atrium. The *azygos vein* which receives segmental veins from the thoracic and posterior abdominal walls (intercostal and lumbar veins) joins the superior vena cava.

Right phrenic nerve

The right and left phrenic nerves are formed in the *cervical plexus* (C3, 4, 5). Besides supplying the diaphragm they give sensory innervation to pleura, pericardium and peritoneum. The thoracic part of the right phrenic nerve reaches the diaphragm lying on the surface of the right brachiocephalic vein, the superior vena cava, the right side of the heart and pericardium (where it lies in front of the root of the lung) and the inferior vena cava.

Right vagus nerve

The right vagus nerve lies on the trachea and crosses behind the root of the lung and breaks up into branches on the oesophagus. It leaves the thorax by passing along with the oesophagus through the diaphragm as the posterior gastric nerve.

Sympathetic trunk

The sympathetic trunks lie on each side of the vertebral column, extending from the base of the skull to the coccyx where the two chains fuse together. Each trunk contains a number of *sympathetic ganglia*, the thoracic region having about 11 ganglia which lie on the neck of the ribs. The ganglia are closely related to the intercostal nerves (Fig. 14.2) from which they receive pre-ganglionic fibres as *white rami communicantes*. The post-ganglionic fibres from the ganglia go back to the intercostal nerves as *grey rami communicantes*. The thoracic ganglia give off the *greater, lesser* and *least splanchnic nerves* to supply the abdominal viscera. The splanchnic nerves are preganglionic fibres which will synapse in collateral ganglia displaced from the sympathetic trunk (e.g. coeliac ganglion) in the abdomen.

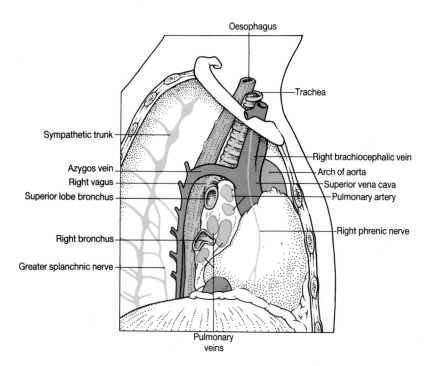

Fig. 14.3 **Mediastinum seen from the right**

Refer to Figures 14.4 and 14.5 and expose the structures on the left side of the mediastinum.

The *ascending aorta* continues upwards and to the left over the root of the left lung as the *arch of the aorta*. It then descends down to become the *descending thoracic aorta*. The arch of the aorta is entirely confined to the superior mediastinum. It has three branches: the *brachiocephalic trunk* (which divides into the right common carotid and the right subclavian arteries), the *left common carotid artery* and the *left subclavian artery*.

Left vagus and left phrenic nerves

Both nerves cross the arch of the aorta; the phrenic nerve descends in front of the root of the lung whereas the vagus crosses behind it. The left vagus gives off an important branch, the *left recurrent laryngeal nerve* as it crosses the arch of the aorta. The left recurrent laryngeal nerve winds round the *ligamentum arteriosus* (Fig. 14.4), a fibrous connection between the left pulmonary artery and the arch of the aorta. The ligamentum arteriosum is the remnant of the *ductus arteriosus* which shunts blood from the pulmonary trunk to the aorta in the fetus. The recurrent laryngeal nerve ascends to the neck lying in the groove between the trachea and the oesophagus and supplies the muscles and mucous membrane of the larynx.

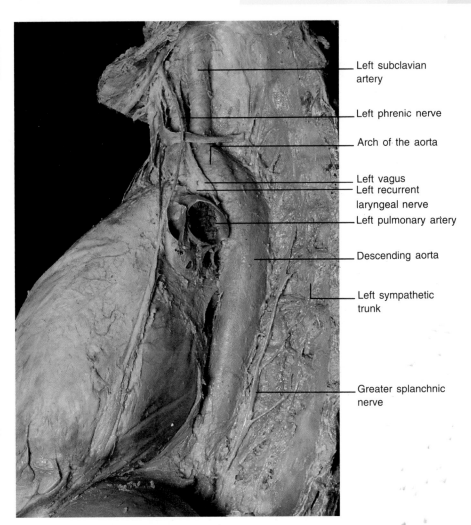

Fig. 14.4 **Left side of the mediastinum**

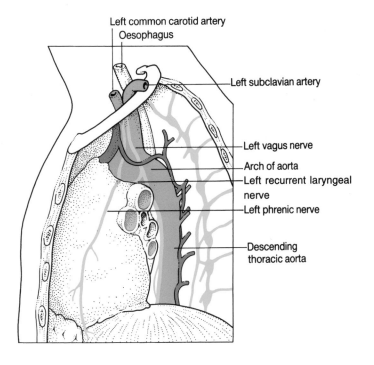

Fig. 14.5 **Mediastinum seen from the left side**

15

The heart and pericardium

The heart is about the size of a clenched fist in the normal individual and lies within the pericardial cavity, in the middle mediastinum. The pericardial cavity is similar in structure and function to the pleural cavity. The pericardium provides for the heart a friction free surface to accommodate its sliding movements.

Components of the pericardium

- The *fibrous pericardium* which is a collagenous outer layer fused with the central tendon of the diaphragm
- The *serous pericardium* consisting of a *parietal layer* which lines the fibrous pericardium and a *visceral layer* which lines the outer surface of the heart and the commencement of the great vessels. The *pericardial cavity* is the space between the parietal and the visceral layers.

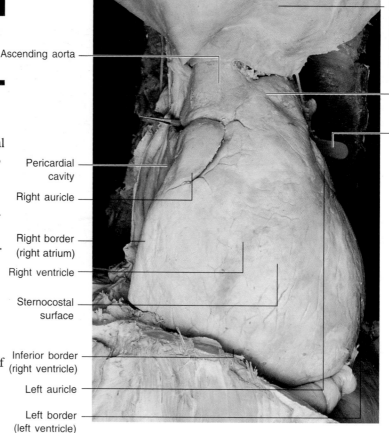

Fig. 15.1 **Anterior aspect of the heart after reflection of fibrous and parietal layer of serous pericardium**

Labels: Ascending aorta; Pericardial cavity; Right auricle; Right border (right atrium); Right ventricle; Sternocostal surface; Inferior border (right ventricle); Left auricle; Left border (left ventricle); Fibrous pericardium and the parietal layer of serous pericardium; Pulmonary trunk; Forceps in the transverse sinus

Transverse and oblique sinuses

Make two vertical and one transverse incisions along the fibrous pericardium and reflect a quadrilateral flap upwards. Refer to Figure 15.1 and identify the layers of the pericardium. Two regions of the pericardial cavity have special names. Define the *ascending aorta* and the *pulmonary trunk* and pass a forceps behind them to define the transverse sinus of the pericardial cavity. Lift up the heart and define the base or posterior surface of the heart formed by the left atrium (Fig. 15.2). The pericardial space behind the *left atrium* is the *oblique sinus*. The oblique sinus separates the left atrium from the oesophagus.

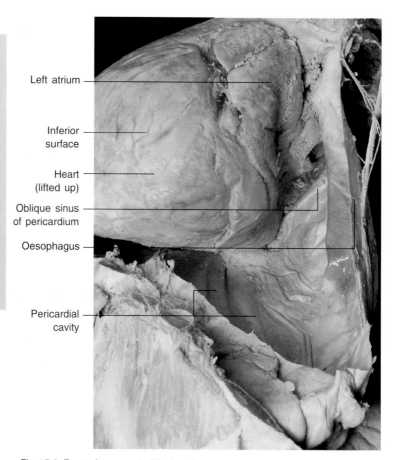

Fig. 15.2 **Posterior aspect of the heart**

Labels: Left atrium; Inferior surface; Heart (lifted up); Oblique sinus of pericardium; Oesophagus; Pericardial cavity

The heart has:

- an anterior or sternocostal surface, formed mostly by the right ventricle
- an inferior or diaphragmatic surface, formed mostly by the left ventricle
- a base or posterior surface, formed by the left atrium
- an apex, formed entirely by the left ventricle.

The borders of the heart are:

- the right border, formed by the right atrium
- the inferior border, formed by the right ventricle
- the left or obtuse border, formed mostly by the left ventricle with the left auricle at its superior end.

Study the borders and surfaces of the heart in situ (Fig. 15.1) and relate them to the radiograph (Fig. 15.3) of the chest.

Refer to Figure 15.4 and define the surface projection of the heart on your partner's chest. Note the areas where the sound produced by the heart valves are best heard.

Removal of the heart

1. Pass a forceps along the transverse sinus and cut across the ascending aorta and the pulmonary trunk
2. Incise the superior and inferior venae cavae
3. Lift up the heart and identify the four pulmonary veins and the left atrium on the posterior surface
4. Cut the pulmonary veins.

The heart can now be removed by simply incising the pericardium between the transverse and oblique sinuses. Hold the heart in the anatomical position and identify again the borders and surfaces and the chambers forming them. Also, identify the atrioventricular groove running obliquely across the heart separating the atria from the ventricles and at right angles to it the anterior and posterior inter-ventricular grooves separating the right ventricle from the left. These grooves contain the blood vessels supplying the heart.

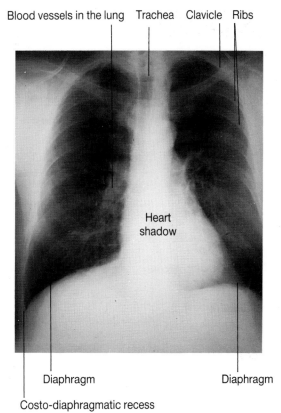

Fig. 15.3 **PA radiograph of the chest**

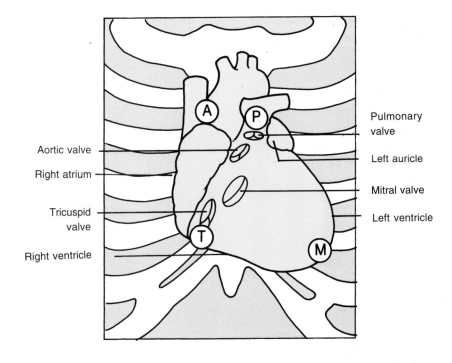

Fig. 15.4 **Surface projections of the heart.** A, P, T and M indicate auscultation areas for the aortic, pulmonary, tricuspid and mitral valves

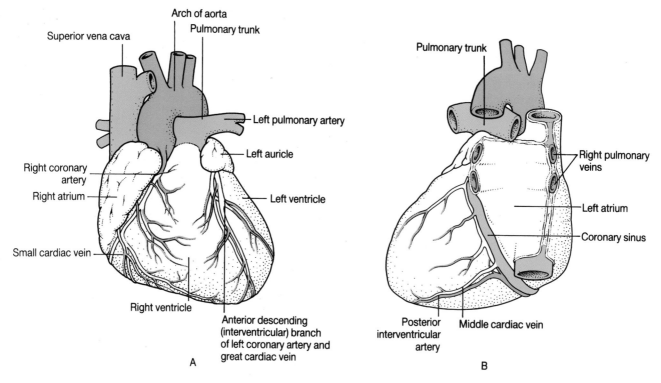

Fig. 15.5 **Heart and great vessels. A.** Anterior view. **B.** Posterior view

BLOOD SUPPLY OF THE HEART

The heart muscle is supplied by the right and left coronary arteries and is drained by the cardiac veins (Fig. 15.5A&B).

The *right coronary artery* which lies in the atrioventricular groove gives off the following branches:

- an artery to the SA node
- the right marginal artery
- the posterior interventricular artery.

Branches from the left coronary artery are:

- the anterior interventricular artery
- the diagonal artery
- the left marginal artery
- the circumflex artery.

Coronary vessels can be dissected by removing piecemeal the fat covering them with a blunt forceps. Be careful to preserve the cardiac veins accompanying the arteries. Before dissecting the arteries, look into the ascending aorta and identify the three aortic sinuses which are depressions alongside the cusps of the aortic valves.

Dissection of the coronary arteries and the cardiac veins

1. Insert a probe into the opening of the right coronary artery from the right (anterior) coronary sinus. Feel for the tip of the probe to the left of the right auricle
2. Expose the right coronary artery in the atrioventricular groove. Trace the artery to the inferior border and then to the diaphragmatic surface where the artery descends as the *posterior interventricular artery.* Trace the *marginal artery*, a branch of the right coronary, along the inferior margin
3. Follow the left coronary artery after probing its opening into the left aortic sinus. The artery lies between the left auricle and the pulmonary trunk. Trace the *anterior interventricular branch* lying in the anterior interventricular groove to

the apex and beyond it to the diaphragmatic surface. Trace the *circumflex branch* to the left margin and then to the diaphragmatic surface.

Cardiac veins can be seen accompanying the arteries. Most of them are tributaries of the *coronary sinus* (Fig. 15.5), a sizeable vein lying in the posterior part of the atrioventricular groove and opening into the right atrium. Identify:

- *the great cardiac vein* accompanying the anterior interventricular artery
- *the middle cardiac vein* along the posterior interventricular artery
- *the small cardiac vein* accompanying the marginal artery.

✳ Angina pectoris is a clinical condition where the chest pain is caused by transient ischaemia of the myocardium resulting from narrowing of the coronary arteries. Myocardial infarction is caused by occlusion of the coronary artery and necrosis of part of the myocardium.

INTERIOR OF THE CHAMBERS

Right atrium

Open the right atrium by making an incision on its anterior wall extending from the right side of the superior vena cava to the right side of the inferior vena cava. Open the atrium, remove blood clots and wash the area thoroughly with cold water and study the following internal features (Figs 15.6 & 15.7):

- the smooth and rough parts of the atrium separated by a vertical ridge, the *crista terminalis*
- the *superior* and *inferior venae cavae* which bring systemic venous blood into the smooth part of the atrium
- the opening of the *coronary sinus* anterior to the opening of the inferior vena cava
- the *fossa ovalis*, an oval depression on the interatrial wall. It is the remnant of the *foramen ovale* in the fetus.

In the fetus, oxygenated blood from the placenta coming through the inferior vena cava passes from the right atrium to the left atrium through the foramen ovale. The interatrial septum is developed from the overlapping septa, the septum primum forming the lower part and the septum secundum (to the right of septum primum) the upper part. Before birth because of the increased pressure in the right atrium, the thin and flexible septum balloons to the left opening a channel between the two septa — the foramen ovale. After birth pressure in the left atrium becomes greater than that in the right and the septum primum is forced against the rigid septum secundum closing the foramen ovale. The lower edge of the septum secundum can be seen as a crescentic edge (limbus fossa ovalis) along the upper part of the fossa ovalis.

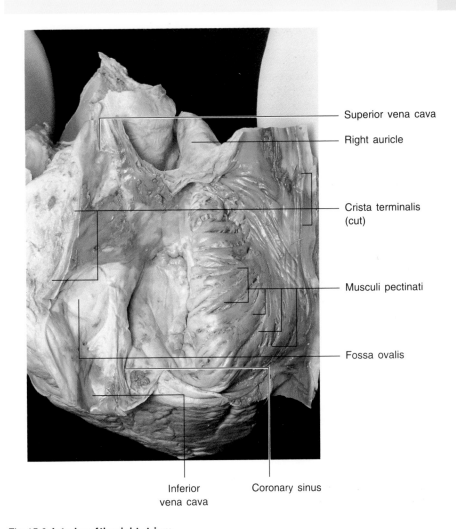

Superior vena cava

Right auricle

Crista terminalis (cut)

Musculi pectinati

Fossa ovalis

Inferior vena cava

Coronary sinus

Fig. 15.6 **Interior of the right atrium**

Right ventricle (Figs 15.7 & 15.8)

Open the right ventricle by continuing the incision from the inferior vena cava along the inferior border of the ventricle to the apex of the heart and from there to the pulmonary trunk. Clean the cavity and define the following:

- the tricuspid orifice and the anterior, posterior and septal cusps of the *tricuspid valve*
- muscular ridges known as *trabeculae carneae*
- the anterior, posterior and septal (small) *papillary muscles* and the *chordae tendineae*. The chordae tendineae connect the papillary muscles to the tricuspid valve cusps. These prevent eversion of the cusps into the atrium during ventricular contraction
- The *septomarginal trabecula* (*moderator band*), a muscular ridge extending from the interventricular septum to the base of the anterior papillary muscle of the heart. The moderator band is a part of the *conducting system* of the heart which regulates the cardiac cycle
- The infundibulum, orifice of the *pulmonary trunk* and the three semilunar cusps of the *pulmonary valve*.

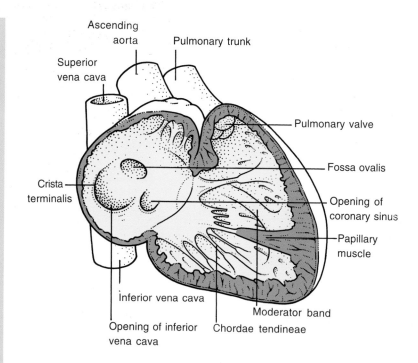

Fig. 15.7 **Interior of the right side of the heart**

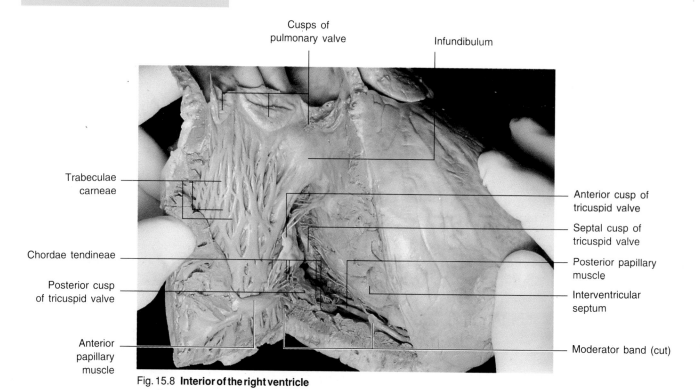

Fig. 15.8 **Interior of the right ventricle**

Left atrium (Fig. 15.9)

Open the left atrium by a vertical incision in the middle of its wall between the two pulmonary veins of each side. Remove the blood clot and observe the following:

- The openings of the four *pulmonary veins*
- The mitral orifice between the left atrium and the left ventricle.

Left ventricle (Figs 15.9 & 15.10)

Open the left ventricle by making an incision along the left border of the ventricle to the apex, following this up to the base of the ascending aorta and along the length of the aorta. Open the ventricle and the aorta, remove the contents, and observe:

- the mitral orifice and the anterior and posterior cusps of the *mitral valve*. The large anterior cusp lies between the aortic and mitral orifices
- the trabeculae carneae
- the papillary muscles and chordae tendineae
- the aortic orifice and the three semilunar *aortic valve* cusps
- the muscular and the membranous parts of the *interventricular septum*. The septum bulges into the right ventricle
- the difference in thickness of the ventricular walls. The right ventricular wall is only about a third of the left ventricular wall.

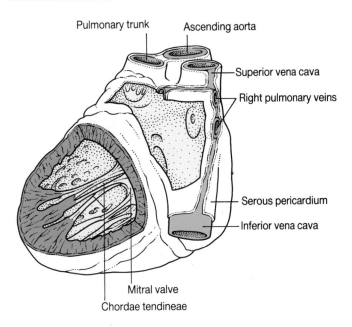

Pulmonary trunk · Ascending aorta · Superior vena cava · Right pulmonary veins · Serous pericardium · Inferior vena cava · Mitral valve · Chordae tendineae

Fig. 15.9 **Interior of the left side of the heart**

Examine the interventricular septum. In the anatomical position it lies almost horizontally with the right ventricle in front of it and the left ventricle behind. Its muscle wall is as thick as that of the left ventricle and it bulges forward into the cavity of the right ventricle. The upper membranous part is fibrous and is thinner.

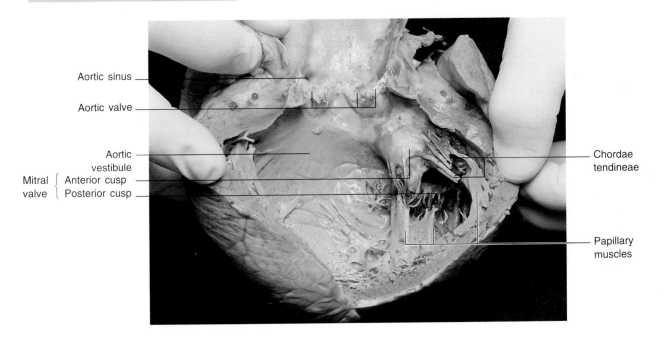

Aortic sinus · Aortic valve · Aortic vestibule · Mitral valve { Anterior cusp / Posterior cusp · Chordae tendineae · Papillary muscles

Fig. 15.10 **Interior of the left ventricle**

16

The superior and posterior mediastinum

Many of the structures in the superior and posterior mediastinum have been exposed in Section 14. In this session we shall review them and also examine some of the deeper structures.

Arch of the aorta

Examine the arch of the aorta and its branches (Fig. 16.1). Note that the left vagus and the left phrenic nerves cross the arch of the aorta. The vein lying across the arch of the aorta is the *left superior intercostal vein*. This drains the second and third left intercostal spaces and in turn drains into the left brachiocephalic vein. Identify the *left recurrent laryngeal nerve* and note that it winds round the *ligamentum arteriosum*. Also examine the remains of the *pulmonary trunk* and its branches.

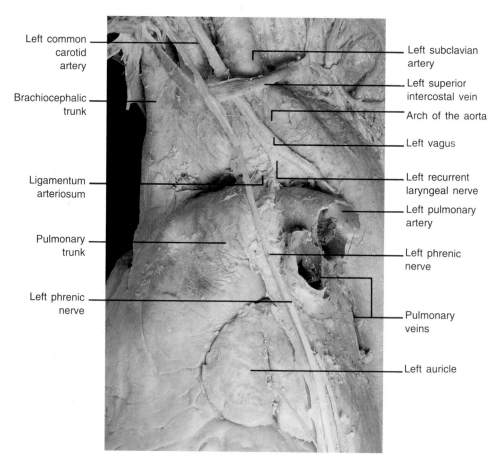

Fig. 16.1 **Arch of the aorta and its branches**

Trachea

The trachea extends from the lower border of the cricoid cartilage in the neck to the tracheal bifurcation at the level of the lower border of the T4 vertebra. In the living, in the erect posture, tracheal bifurcation is at a lower level. The trachea is made up of a series of C-shaped cartilages closed posteriorly by the trachealis muscle. The trachea is elastic enabling it to stretch during swallowing. Its diameter also changes during coughing. The cervical part of the trachea lies in the midline and is easily palpable.

The angle of bifurcation of the trachea in the adult is such that the right main bronchus is more vertical than the left. The cartilage at the tracheal bifurcation is the keel-shaped *carina* which projects into the lumen as a vertical ridge. Flattening of this ridge is a sign of alteration of the bifurcation angle, often due to enlargement of the tracheobroncheal group of lymph nodes. The angle of bifurcation of the trachea is normally wider in children, with no difference in the angulation of the right and left main bronchi.

Remove the remains of the pericardium and the pulmonary veins and also the pulmonary trunk and its branches and expose the trachea and the right and left main bronchi. Examine the relations of the trachea. Note that the arch of the aorta as it hooks over the left main bronchus lies on the anterior and left surfaces of the trachea (Fig. 16.2). The oesophagus lies behind the trachea.

Clean the oesophagus and the descending aorta (Fig. 16.2). Note the oesophageal plexus of nerves contributed by the right and left vagus nerves.

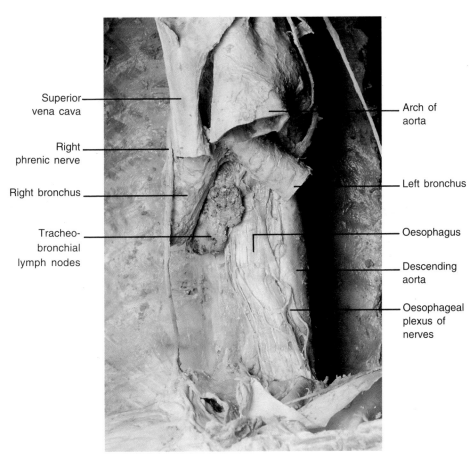

Fig. 16.2 **Superior and posterior mediastinum**

Oesophagus

The oesophagus starts as a continuation of the pharynx at the level of C6 vertebra and ends by entering the stomach at the cardiac orifice. The thoracic part of the oesophagus lies in the superior and posterior mediastinum and enters the abdomen by piercing the diaphragm. In the superior mediastinum it lies behind the trachea with the arch of the aorta lying on its left side. The left recurrent laryngeal nerve lies in the groove between the trachea and the oesophagus. The left main bronchus crosses in front of the oesophagus and the part below that is related to the left atrium. The arch of the aorta, the left main bronchus and the left atrium produce indentations on the oesophagus which can be seen clearly on radiograph taken after barium swallow (Fig. 16.3).

> ✳ Enlargement of the left atrium, as occurs in stenosis of the mitral valve, can produce difficulty in swallowing and an obvious narrowing of the oesophagus on barium swallow.

The oesophagus lies to the right of the *descending aorta* (continuation of the arch of the aorta). It crosses in front of the descending aorta as it leaves the thorax (Fig. 16.2).

> Clean the descending aorta and identify the posterior intercostal arteries branching off it. On the right side of the lower end of the oesophagus find the thoracic duct and trace it upwards.

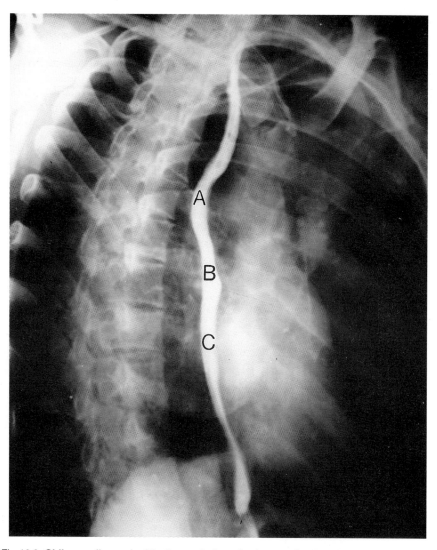

Fig. 16.3 **Oblique radiograph of the thorax during a 'barium swallow' outlining the oesophagus.** The three indentations produced by the arch of the aorta (A), left bronchus (B) and the left atrium (C) are seen well

The descending (thoracic) aorta commences where the arch of the aorta ends at the lower border of T4 vertebra. It leaves the posterior mediastinum in the midline at the level of T12 vertebra by passing between the crura of the diaphragm. The descending aorta gives off nine pairs of posterior intercostal arteries, a pair of subcostal arteries, two bronchial arteries for the left lung and some small branches to the oesophagus.

> ✳ 'Radicular arteries' arise from the posterior intercostal arteries and supply the spinal cord. One such artery (usually from the 10th or 11th intercostal space) is large and is known as the great radicular artery or artery of Adamkiewicz. Blood flow through radicular arteries may be interfered with during aortic surgery producing ischaemia of the spinal cord resulting in paraplegia.

Thoracic duct

The thoracic duct starts as the continuation of the cysterna chyli in the abdomen. Its course and termination is illustrated in Figure 16.4.

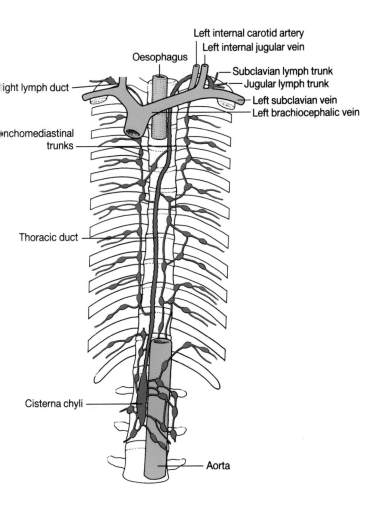

Fig. 16.4 **Cisterna chyli, thoracic duct and right lymph duct**

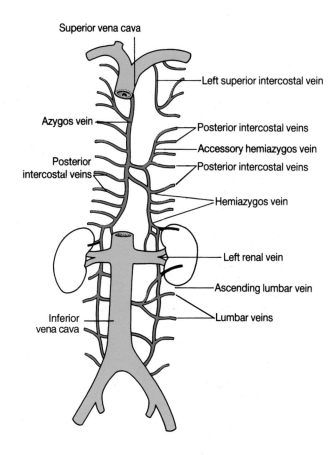

Fig. 16.5 **Veins of the posterior chest and abdominal wall**

Finally clean and trace the azygos vein on the right and the hemiazygos veins on the left and note the connections between them (Fig. 16.5).

The azygos vein enters the thorax through the aortic opening of the diaphragm and passes upwards lying on the vertebral bodies. At the level of T4 vertebra it arches over the root of the right lung to enter the superior vena cava. The azygos vein receives the lower eight posterior intercostal veins of the right side and the right superior intercostal vein. The hemiazygos veins which receive the intercostal veins of the left side drain into the azygos vein.

THE
ABDOMEN

17

The abdominal wall and inguinal canal

OSTEOLOGY AND SURFACE ANATOMY

Refer to Figure 17.1 and identify the following landmarks on the skeleton:

- the lower costal margin
- the xiphisternum
- the anterior superior iliac spine and iliac crest
- the pubic tubercle, pubic crest and pubic symphysis.

Palpate these bony landmarks on yourself or on your partner

Skin reflection

Make a vertical incision extending from the xiphoid process to the pubic symphysis and another incision from the pubic symphysis to the anterior superior iliac spine extending it backwards along the iliac crest. Reflect the skin from the anterior and lateral aspect of the abdomen.

The *superficial fascia* in the anterior abdominal wall has a superficial fatty layer and a deeper membranous layer. It contains the *lateral* and *anterior cutaneous branches* of the *lower intercostal nerves and vessels*, the dissection of which is difficult and time consuming.

Refer to Figures 17.2 and 17.3 and clean the *external oblique* muscle. Note that the muscle is fleshy laterally and posteriorly and forms an *aponeurosis* anteriorly contributing to the sheath covering the rectus abdominis muscle. Identify the lower border of the muscle, the inguinal ligament. Note that the *inguinal ligament* extends from the anterior superior iliac spine to the pubic tubercle. Above and medial to the pubic tubercle clean the *superficial inguinal ring* which transmits the *spermatic cord* in the male and the *round ligament of the uterus* in the female.

Cut through the external oblique and reflect a quadrilateral flap forward as in Figure 17.4 to expose the *internal oblique*.

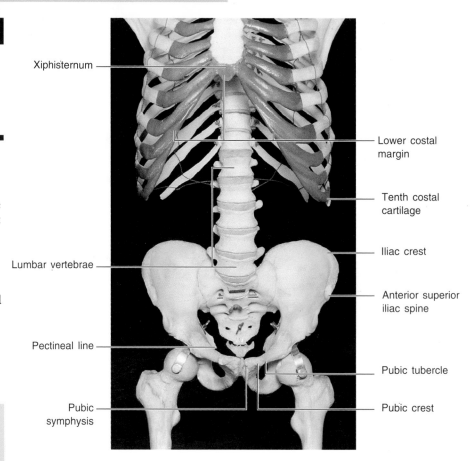

Fig. 17.1 **Bony thoracic cage and the pelvis**

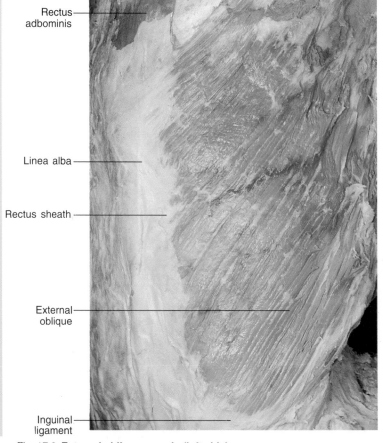

Fig. 17.2 **External oblique muscle (left side)**

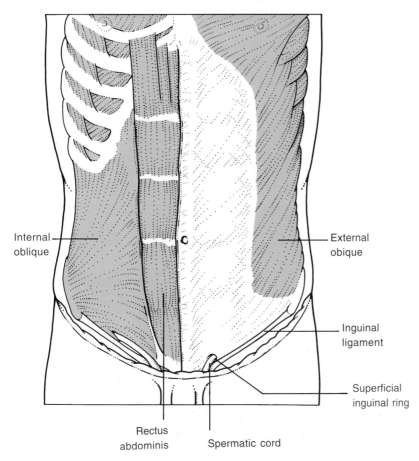

Internal oblique

External obique

Inguinal ligament

Superficial inguinal ring

Rectus abdominis

Spermatic cord

Fig. 17.3 **Muscles of the anterior abdominal wall: anterior view**

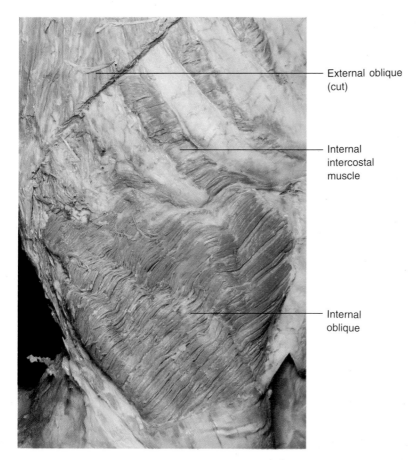

External oblique (cut)

Internal intercostal muscle

Internal oblique

Fig. 17.4 **Internal oblique muscle (right side)**

Cut a similar flap for the internal oblique to expose the *transversus* (Fig. 17.5). Identify the trunks of the *intercostal nerves* between the internal oblique and the transversus.

In the male examine the *spermatic cord* and note that the lower fibres of the internal oblique cross in front of the spermatic cord and that some of the fibres continue on to the cord as the *cremaster muscle* (Fig. 17.6). Also note that the lower part of the internal oblique and transversus fuse together as they lie above the cord and form the *conjoint tendon*. The conjoint tendon lies behind the spermatic cord and is inserted into the pubic crest and the *pectineal line* of the hip bone (Fig. 17.1).

Carefully cut through the lateral part of the conjoint tendon and expose the transversalis fascia deep to it. Identify the *deep inguinal ring* (Fig. 17.6) which is the point where the transversalis fascia is invaginated by the spermatic cord. The deep inguinal ring lies just above the *midinguinal point* which is the midpoint of a line connecting the anterior superior iliac spine and the pubic symphysis. You will notice an artery lying *medial* to the deep inguinal ring. This is the *inferior epigastric artery*, a branch of the external iliac artery. The inferior epigastric artery enters the rectus sheath and anastomoses with the superior epigastric artery (see below).

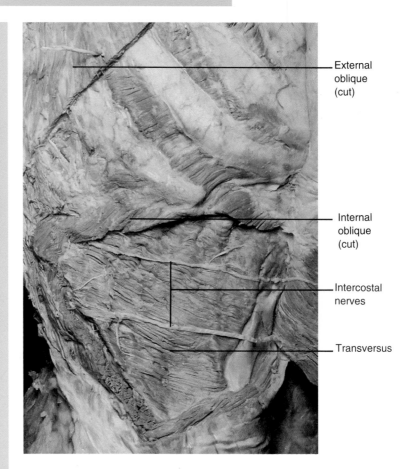

External oblique (cut)

Internal oblique (cut)

Intercostal nerves

Transversus

Fig. 17.5 **Transversus muscle (right side)**

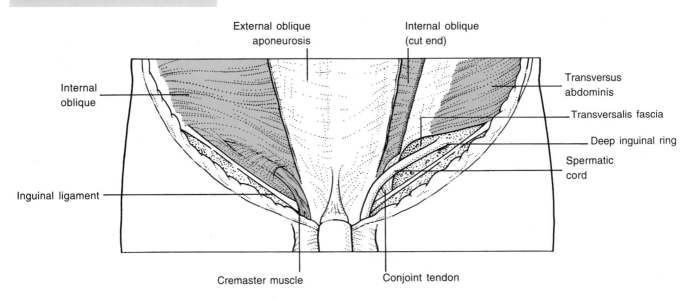

External oblique aponeurosis

Internal oblique (cut end)

Transversus abdominis

Transversalis fascia

Deep inguinal ring

Spermatic cord

Internal oblique

Inguinal ligament

Cremaster muscle

Conjoint tendon

Fig. 17.6 **Inguinal region in the male.** On the right-hand side of the inguinal region the external oblique has been removed; on the left-hand side the external oblique and internal oblique have been partially removed

Inguinal canal

The *inguinal canal* is a slit-like space in between the muscles of the anterior abdominal wall, above the medial half of the inguinal ligament. It contains the *spermatic cord* and the *ilioinguinal nerve* in the male and the *round ligament of the uterus* and the *ilioinguinal nerve* in the female. It is about 6 cm long and extends from the *deep inguinal ring* (in the transversalis fascia) to the *superficial inguinal ring* (in the external oblique aponeurosis).

Walls of the inguinal canal. The anterior wall (i.e. structures in front of the spermatic cord) is formed by the external oblique aponeurosis reinforced laterally by fibres of the internal oblique. The posterior wall (structures behind the spermatic cord) is formed throughout by the transversalis fascia and is reinforced medially by the conjoint tendon. The roof of the canal (structures above the cord) is formed by the arched fibres of the transversus and the internal oblique. The floor is formed by the inguinal ligament and its continuation on to the pectineal line, the *lacunar ligament.*

> ✳ **Inguinal hernias**
> Part of the intestine or peritoneal fold can herniate through the inguinal canal as an *inguinal hernia.* These hernias are more common in the male as the canal is bigger. An *indirect inguinal hernia* comes through the deep inguinal ring and hence traverses the whole extent of the canal. *It is contained inside the coverings of the spermatic cord. A direct inguinal hernia* on the other hand invaginates the posterior wall of the canal.

Rectus abdominis and the rectus sheath

The aponeuroses of the external oblique, internal oblique and the transversus form the *rectus sheath.* Medial to the rectus the aponeuroses of both sides fuse in the midline to form the *linea alba.* The rectus abdominis muscle extends vertically upwards from the pubic crest to the lower costal margin.

Study the formation of the rectus sheath by referring to Figure 17.7. Note that below halfway between the pubic symphysis and the umbilicus, all three aponeuroses cross in front of the rectus abdominis. Thus the posterior wall of the sheath is formed only by the transversalis fascia. Above that level the external oblique contributes to the front of the rectus sheath, the transversus to its back and the internal oblique splits, one layer going in front and the other behind (Fig. 17.8).

> Incise the anterior wall of the rectus sheath and expose its contents. Note that the anterior layer is adherent to three *tendinous intersections* of the rectus abdominis. The sheath contains the *rectus abdominis,* the *pyramidalis* muscle (a small muscle in the lower part), the *lower five intercostal nerves* and the *subcostal nerve* with the accompanying vessels and the *superior and inferior epigastric arteries and veins.*

The anastomosis between the superior and inferior epigastric arteries provides a collateral circulation between the subclavian and the external iliac arteries. This collateral channel will enlarge in coarctation of the aorta or any other condition narrowing the aorta beyond the origin of the subclavian artery.

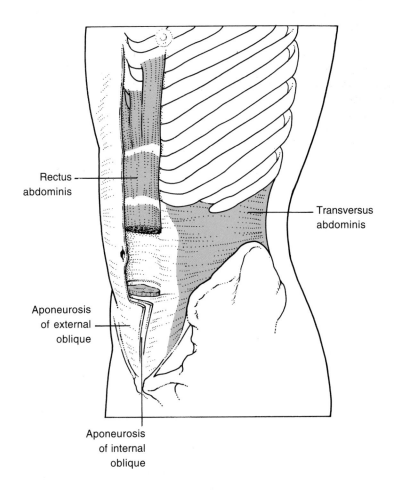

Rectus abdominis

Transversus abdominis

Aponeurosis of external oblique

Aponeurosis of internal oblique

Fig. 17.7 **Rectus abdominis and the rectus sheath: oblique view.** Note that in the lower part all three aponeuroses lie in front of the rectus

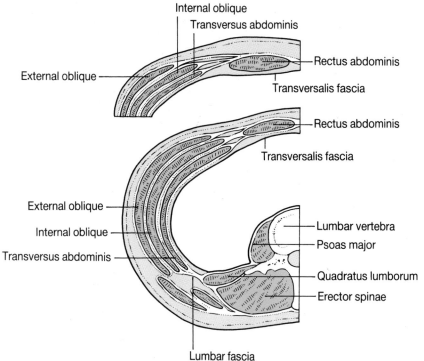

Fig. 17.8 **Transverse section of the abdominal wall, showing the arrangement of muscles, lumbar fascia and rectus sheath.** The insert shows the rectus abdominis and the formation of the rectus sheath below the arcuate line.

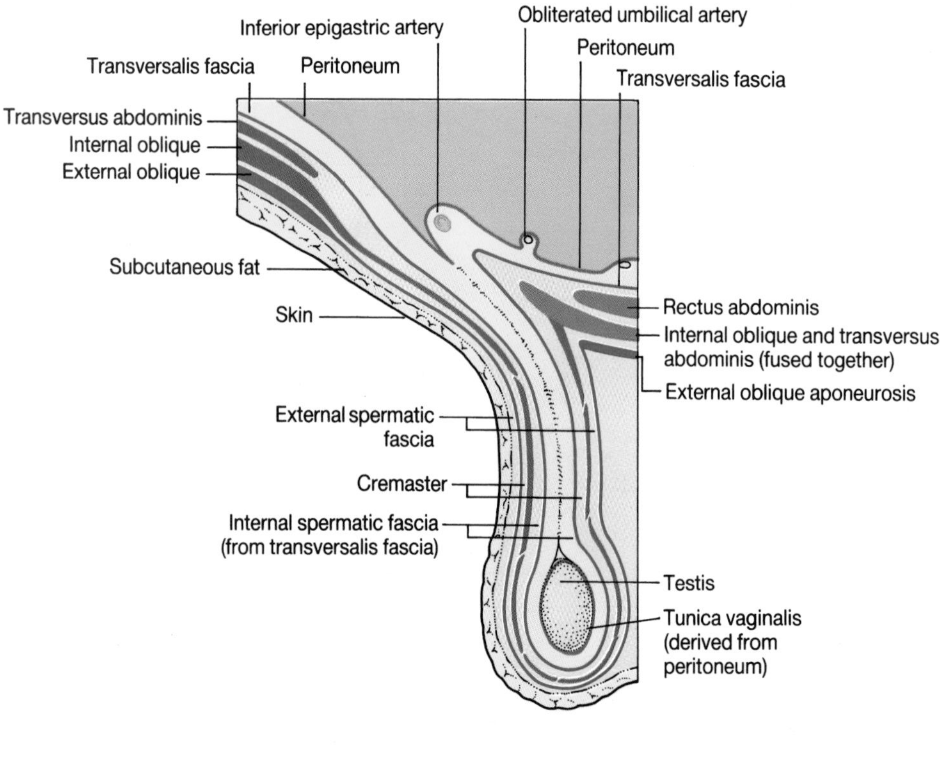

✳ A paramedian incision — an incision slightly lateral to the midline — is usually used by surgeons to gain access to the abdominal cavity. After incising the skin the superficial fascia and the anterior layer of the rectus sheath, the rectus abdominis is retracted laterally to avoid traction on the nerves (the intercostal nerves and the subcostal nerve enter the muscles from its lateral aspect). The posterior layer of the rectus sheath along with the transversalis fascia and the underlying peritoneum is then cut to enter the cavity of the abdomen.

Nerve supply of the anterior abdominal wall muscles

The rectus abdominis and the external oblique are supplied by nerves T7–T12 (lower five intercostal nerves and the subcostal nerve) and the internal oblique and the transversus by the same nerves with the addition of L1. L1 supplies the lower fibres of the internal oblique and the transversus forming the conjoint tendon which maintains the integrity of the inguinal canal.

Scrotum, testis and the spermatic cord (Fig. 17.9)

The following dissection will expose the testis and the spermatic cord and their coverings.

Make an incision downwards from the pubic tubercle and reflect the skin of the scrotum. The superficial fascia of the scrotum has a thin layer of muscle — the dartos muscle. Remove the dartos muscle and expose the *external spermatic fascia* which is a continuation of the aponeurosis of the external oblique. Next attempt to define the cremaster muscle and fascia (a continuation of the internal oblique) and the internal spermatic fascia (continuation of the transversalis fascia). Remove these coverings and identify the *ductus (vas) deferens*, which has a thick wall, the testicular artery and the pampiniform plexus of veins. Incise the *tunica vaginalis*, the peritoneum covering the testis and the epididymis. Trace the ductus to the lower pole of the testis where it becomes continuous with the epididymis. Examine the testis and the epididymis.

Fig. 17.9 **Schematic diagram of the inguinal canal, and the coverings of testis and spermatic cord**

The epididymis lies posterior to the testis. Its upper part is known as the head of the epididymis (Fig. 17.10) and its lower part continues as the ductus. Sperms produced in the seminiferous tubules of the testis are stored in the epididymis and the ductus before ejaculation. The ductus deferens which joins the prostatic part of the urethra transport sperms to the urethra.

The ductus deferens joins the duct of the seminal vesicle to form the ejaculatory duct. The ejaculatory duct joins the prostatic part of the urethra. The ductus deferens transports sperms to the urethra.

The testis is supplied by the testicular artery, a branch of the abdominal artery and is drained by the *pampiniform plexus* of veins. The testicular artery also supplies the epididymis. Pampiniform plexus of veins join together to form a single testicular vein at the deep inguinal ring. On the left side the testicular vein drains into the left renal vein and on the right side into the inferior vena cava. The lymphatics of the testis drain into the paraaortic nodes which lie along the aorta at this level of the origin of the testicular arteries.

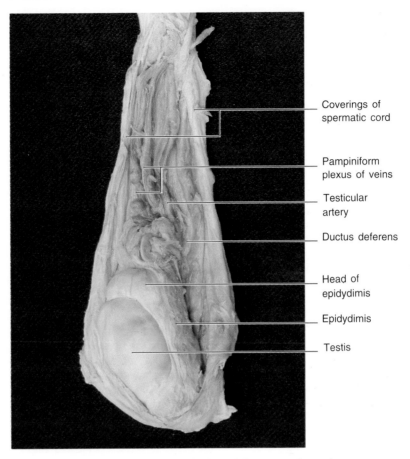

Coverings of spermatic cord

Pampiniform plexus of veins

Testicular artery

Ductus deferens

Head of epidydimis

Epidydimis

Testis

Fig. 17.10 **Dissection of testis, epididymis and the spermatic cord**

18

The peritoneal cavity

The abdominal cavity is lined by peritoneum. The *peritoneal cavity* of the abdomen is a potential space between the *parietal* and the *visceral* layers of peritoneum. The *parietal peritoneum* lines the inner surface of the abdominal and pelvic wall. The *visceral peritoneum* is the continuation of the parietal peritoneum and it invests many of the abdominal organs. In some, such as duodenum, ascending and descending colon and kidneys, only the anterior surfaces of the organs are covered by the peritoneum making them *retroperitoneal organs*. Peritoneal membranes connecting the parietal peritoneum to the visceral peritoneum have different names in different regions. The *mesentery* connects the small intestine, *mesocolon* the large intestine, *omentum* is attached to the stomach, and the peritoneal *ligaments* connect the liver.

Open the peritoneal cavity by making a vertical and a transverse incision. Turn back the flaps and note that the abdominal wall is lined by the parietal peritoneum.

In the upper right flap identify the *falciform ligament* extending onto the liver (Fig. 18.1). Feel the cord-like *ligamentum teres* (obliterated umbilical vein) in its free edge. Trace the falciform ligament to the liver. The liver is divided into right and left lobes by the falciform ligament. Insert your hand over the right lobe of the liver, push your hand between the liver and the diaphragm and feel the superior layer of the *coronary ligament*. Similarly, insert your hand under the right lobe of the liver and push it upwards between the posterior surface of the liver and the diaphragm and feel the inferior layer of the coronary ligament. You will be able to appreciate that the right layer of the falciform ligament continues as the peritoneum covering the right lobe of the liver and gets reflected onto the diaphragm as the superior and inferior layers of the

coronary ligament. The right edge of the coronary ligament is known as the *right triangular ligament.*

Now trace the left layer of the falciform ligament to the left lobe of the liver and note that after enclosing the left lobe it is reflected onto the diaphragm as the *left triangular ligament.* You may be able to see the left triangular ligament connecting the left lobe to the diaphragm if the liver is gently pulled downwards.

Gently lift up the left lobe of the liver to expose the stomach and the *lesser omentum.* Note that the lesser omentum extends from the liver to the *lesser curvature* of the stomach and to the first part of the duodenum (Figs 18.2 & 18.3). Define the right *free border* of the lesser omentum. Palpate the structures in the free border. It contains the *common bile duct*, the *hepatic artery* and the *portal vein.* Pass your finger behind the free edge of the lesser omentum through the *epiploic foramen* into the *lesser sac* of peritoneum.

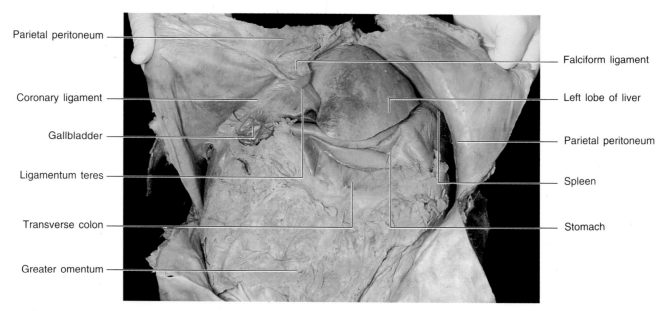

Parietal peritoneum

Coronary ligament

Gallbladder

Ligamentum teres

Transverse colon

Greater omentum

Falciform ligament

Left lobe of liver

Parietal peritoneum

Spleen

Stomach

Fig. 18.1 **Upper part of the peritoneal cavity**

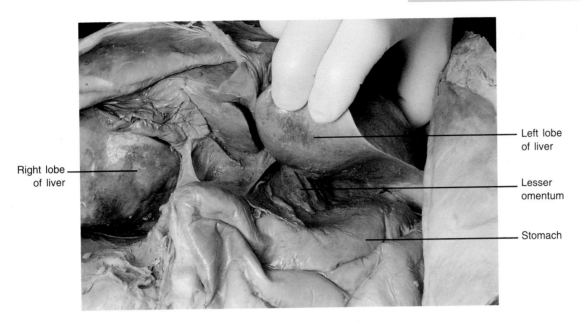

Right lobe of liver

Left lobe of liver

Lesser omentum

Stomach

Fig. 18.2 **Liver, stomach and lesser omentum**

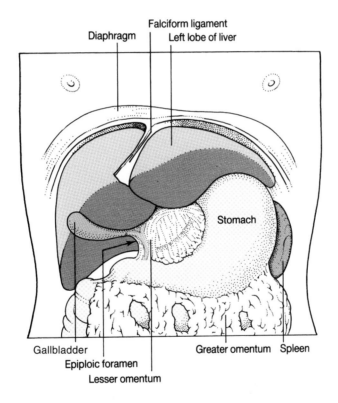

Diaphragm

Falciform ligament
Left lobe of liver

Stomach

Gallbladder

Epiploic foramen

Lesser omentum

Greater omentum   Spleen

Fig. 18.3 **Liver, stomach, lesser omentum and diaphragm: anterior view**

The lesser sac is a part of the peritoneal cavity and lies behind the lesser omentum and the stomach and also extends into the *greater omentum* (Fig. 18.4A&B). The rest of the peritoneal cavity is known as the *greater sac*. The greater sac and the lesser sac communicate with each other through the epiploic foramen (Fig. 18.3).

The greater omentum hangs down like an apron from the greater curvature of the stomach. The transverse colon is attached to its posterior layer (Fig. 18.1). To the left the greater omentum extends as the *gastrosplenic ligament* which splits to invest the spleen and continues onto the left kidney as the *lieno-renal ligament* (Fig. 18.4B).

Define the greater omentum. Insert your hand under the left costal margin and feel the *spleen*. The spleen lies to the left of the stomach. Define the gastrosplenic ligament extending from the stomach to the spleen. Note that it is continuous with the greater omentum. Insert your hand between the spleen and the diaphragm and feel the bulge of the *left kidney* and the lieno-renal ligament.

Lift up the greater omentum and the transverse colon. Define the *transverse mesocolon* attaching the latter to the posterior abdominal wall (Fig. 18.5 & 18.6). Also identify the coils of *jejunum* and *ileum* and the *mesentery*. Verify the line of attachment of the mesentery to the posterior abdominal wall. This is known as the *root of the mesentery*. The duodenum which extends between the stomach and the jejunum is retroperitoneal and is not visible at this stage. Identify by palpation the junction between the duodenum and the jejunum, the *duodenojejunal flexure*.

Trace the ileum to the *ileo-caecal* junction. Look for the *vermiform appendix* and its mesentery. Identify the *ascending* and the *descending colon*. Note the longitudinal bands of smooth muscle on the colon, these are the *taenia coli*. Trace the descending colon to the pelvis where it becomes the *sigmoid colon* which then continues as the *rectum*. Identify the sigmoid *mesocolon*, the peritoneal membrane connecting the sigmoid colon to the abdominal and pelvic wall.

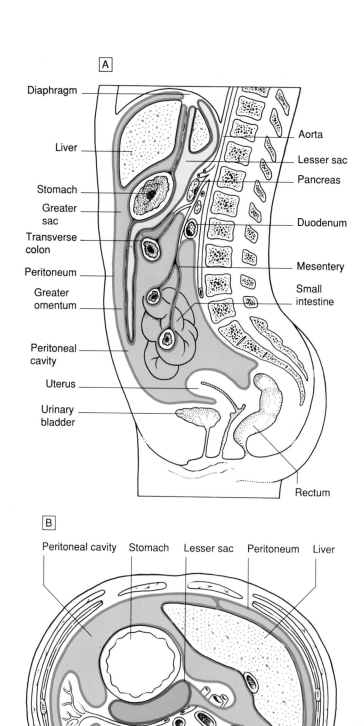

Fig. 18.4 **Peritoneum and peritoneal cavity. A.** Midline sagittal section. **B.** Transverse section at the level of vertebra T12

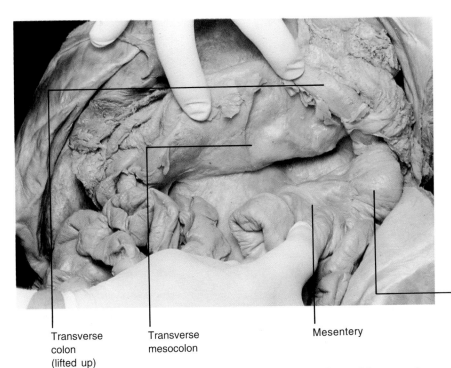

In the male identify the upper surface of the *urinary bladder*. The peritoneal space between the bladder and the rectum is the *recto-vesical pouch* and is the most dependent part of the peritoneal cavity.

In the female identify the *uterus*. The peritoneal space between the rectum and the uterus is the *recto-uterine pouch* and this is the lowermost part of the peritoneal cavity in the female. The peritoneal space between the uterus and the urinary bladder is the *utero-vesical pouch*.

Small intestine

Transverse colon (lifted up)

Transverse mesocolon

Mesentery

Fig. 18.5 **Transverse colon, transverse mesocolon, small intestine and the mesentery**

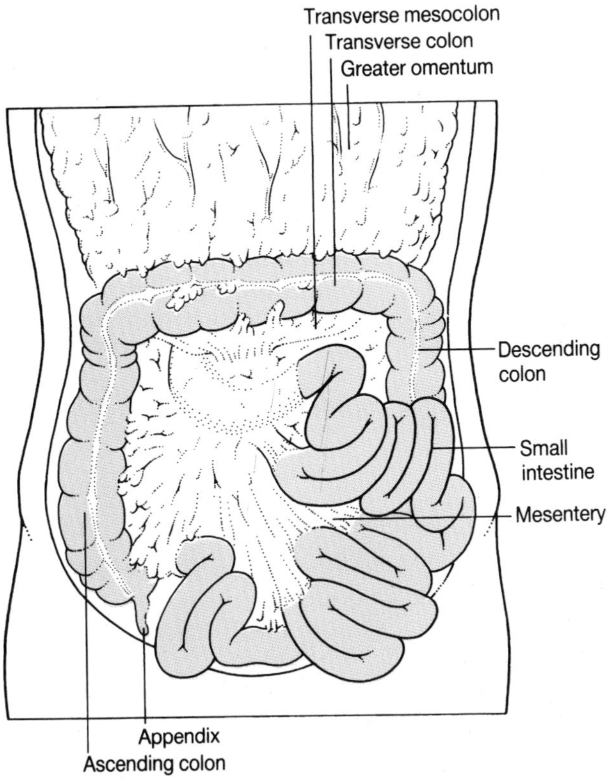

Transverse mesocolon
Transverse colon
Greater omentum

Descending colon

Small intestine

Mesentery

Appendix
Ascending colon

Fig. 18.6 **Abdominal contents seen after lifting up the greater omen**

19

The liver gallbladder and stomach

This dissection will examine the gross features of the liver and gallbladder, the formation of the common bile duct, and the gross features of the stomach as well as its blood supply.

Liver

The liver occupies a major part of the upper abdominal cavity. It is supplied by the *hepatic artery* and the *hepatic portal vein* and is drained by the *hepatic veins* which joins the *inferior vena cava*. Bile produced by the liver is drained by the right and left *hepatic ducts* which join to form the *common hepatic duct*. This is joined by the *cystic duct* from the gallbladder to form the *common bile duct* (Fig. 19.1). The common bile duct which lies in the free border of the lesser omentum eventually drains into the second part of the duodenum after crossing behind the first part of the duodenum and the head of the pancreas.

✳ Variation in the pattern of the biliary duct system is common. The cystic duct may join the right hepatic duct or the lower part of the common bile duct. Failure to appreciate these variations may result in errors in gallbladder surgery.

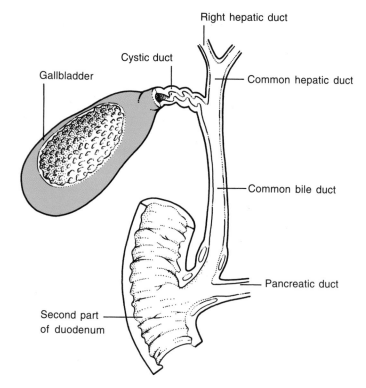

Fig. 19.1 **Biliary system**

Pull the liver upwards to expose again the lesser omentum and identify its free border forming the anterior boundary of the epiploic foramen. Palpate in its free border the *common bile duct*, the *hepatic artery* and the *portal vein*. Expose them by peeling off the peritoneum with a forceps (Fig. 19.2). Cut these structures and you will be able to see, or at least feel, the inferior vena cava which forms the

posterior boundary of the epiploic foramen. Cut the inferior vena cava as close to the liver as possible.

Identify again the falciform ligament, the coronary ligament and the left triangular ligament which connects the liver to the diaphragm . Cut these ligaments. Gently push the liver downwards and make another cut on the inferior vena cava, just below the diaphragm, and remove the liver.

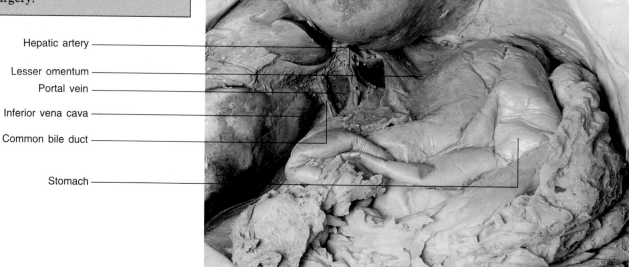

Fig. 19.2 **Structures bounding the epiploic foramen**

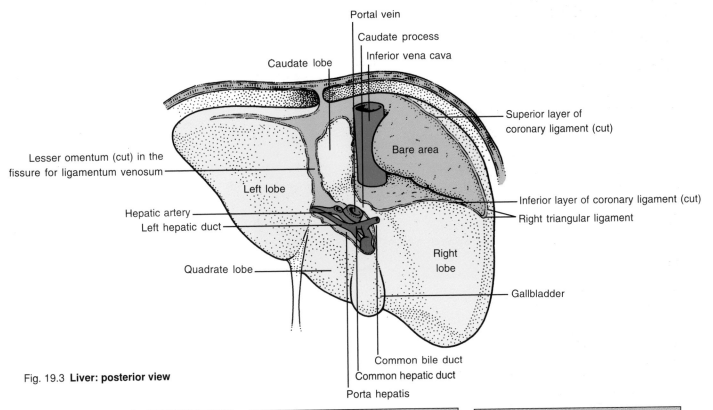

Fig. 19.3 **Liver: posterior view**

Examine the posterior and the inferior surfaces of the liver (Fig. 19.3). Identify the *caudate* and *quadrate* lobes, the *fissure for the ligamentum venosum* and the cut edge of the lesser omentum. Also identify the areas related to the stomach, the right kidney and the hepatic flexure of the colon. Open the inferior vena cava and note the openings of the hepatic veins. The area to the right of the inferior vena cava, devoid of peritoneum, is the *bare area* of the liver. The two layers of the coronary ligaments and the inferior vena cava bound the bare area.

The *porta hepatis* is the area on the inferior surface containing the hepatic artery, bile duct and the hepatic portal vein.

Define the structures in the porta hepatis. Clean the right and left hepatic ducts and note that they join to form the common hepatic duct. Similarly define the right and left branches of the common hepatic artery and the two branches of the hepatic portal vein.

Define the gallbladder and the cystic duct. Note how the common bile duct is formed (Fig. 19.1). Find the *cystic artery* which supplies the gallbladder. This is usually a branch of the right hepatic artery but may have a variable origin.

✳ The liver is normally not palpable, except in infants and in those with a thin abdominal wall. The liver is palpated by feeling for its sharp inferior margin. It descends downwards during inspiration.

Gallbladder

The gallbladder stores and concentrates bile. The *fundus* of the gallbladder is its blind end which projects beyond the inferior surface of the liver. The fundus continues as the *body* of the gallbladder. The junction between the body and the cystic duct is the *neck* of the gallbladder. The gallbladder is not normally palpable. When it is distended due to obstruction of the bile duct, the fundus is palpable at the tip of the right ninth costal cartilage in the midclavicular line.

✳ The gallbladder is liable to recurrent infection, a condition known as *cholecystitis*. The pain in cholecystitis may be initially felt in the epigastrium but may also be felt as a referred pain over the right shoulder. Stones or calculi may occur in the gallbladder and are often associated with infections.

✳ *Cholecystectomy* (removal of the gallbladder). This is a common abdominal operation. After cholecystectomy the hepatic ducts and the bile duct dilate to store bile. Haemorrhage during cholecystectomy may be controlled by compressing the hepatic artery in the free border of the lesser omentum (Pringle's manoeuvre).

Open the gallbladder and examine its interior. Note that the mucosa is thrown into folds giving a honeycomb appearance in the body and fundus. In the neck the mucosal folds are spiral shaped (the spiral valve).

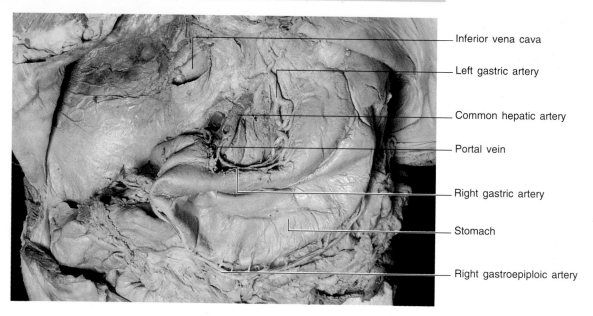

Fig. 19.4 **Blood supply of the stomach**

Stomach

Carefully remove the peritoneum from the lesser curvature of the stomach and demonstrate the left and right gastric arteries (Figs 19.4 & 19.5). Similarly demonstrate the right and left gastroepiploic arteries and the short gastric arteries along the greater curvature of the stomach. Define the *gastroduodenal artery*, a branch of the common hepatic artery lying behind the first part of the duodenum (Fig. 19.5).

Identify the lower end of the oesophagus. Look for the anterior

gastric nerves (from the left vagus) on the anterior surface of the oesophagus. The posterior gastric nerve lies behind the oesophagus.

Identify the *pylorus*. This may be felt as a thickening (the pyloric sphincter) at the junction between the stomach and the duodenum.

Cut through the oesophagus and the first part of the duodenum just beyond the pylorus. Now cut the greater omentum and the gastrosplenic ligament (the continuation of the greater omentum to the left) along the greater

curvature. Cut the arteries on the lesser and greater curvatures and remove the stomach. Note the shape of the stomach and identify the fundus, body and pyloric regions (Fig. 19.5). Open the stomach, wash off the contents, if any, and examine its interior. Note the longitudinal folds of the mucosa, the rugae, near the lesser curvature. Remove the mucosa in the pyloric region and examine the *pyloric sphincter*. Note that the sphincter is formed by thickening of the circular muscle.

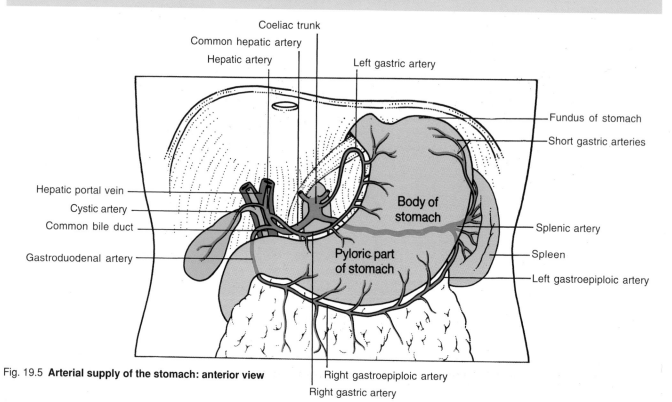

Fig. 19.5 **Arterial supply of the stomach: anterior view**

20

The small and large intestines

Small intestine

The small intestine, the major site of digestion and absorption, extends from the pylorus of the stomach to the ileocaecal junction. It is 2–7 metres long. The first 25 cm is the *duodenum*, the next two-fifths is *jejunum* and the distal three-fifths is the *ileum*. Transition between the jejunum and ileum is gradual. There is no landmark between the two.

The duodenum is C-shaped. It is retroperitoneal and is not mobile unlike the jejunum and ileum. The duodenum will be examined later along with the posterior abdominal wall structures.

Examine the jejunum and ileum. Identify the junction between the duodenum and the jejunum, the *duodenojejunal flexure*. Define the line of attachment of the mesentery — the *root of the mesentery*. It extends obliquely downwards and to the right to the ileocaecal junction. The root of the mesentery is only about 15 cm long.

The arterial supply of the jejunum and ileum is derived from the *superior mesenteric artery*, a branch of the abdominal aorta. The corresponding veins drain into the *superior mesenteric vein* and then into the *hepatic portal vein*. The arterial branches form arcades from which terminal vessels — *vasae rectae* — supply the gut wall (Figs 20.1 & 20.2).

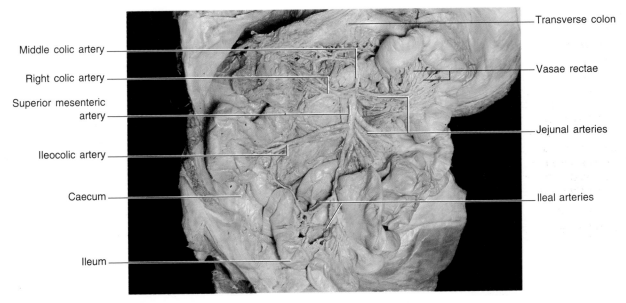

Fig. 20.1 **Superior mesenteric artery**

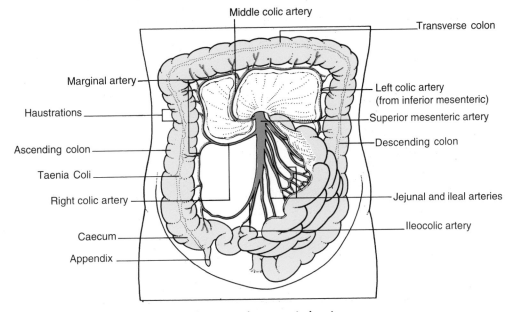

Fig. 20.2 **Distribution of the superior mesenteric artery**

Remove the peritoneum from the surface of the mesentery and expose the blood vessels supplying the jejunum and ileum. Demonstrate the difference in the patterns of the arterial arcades and the vasae rectae (Fig. 20.3). Note that the jejunum has fewer arcades making the vasae rectae longer than those in the ileum.

✳ Loops of small intestine may get twisted around abnormal peritoneal bands or adhesions, producing a *volvulus*. A volvulus can result in intestinal obstruction and strangulation of its blood supply. Malrotation of the gut during development may result in a very short root of the mesentery and this may also produce volvulus.

✳ *Meckel's (ileal) diverticulum.* This is a remnant of the vitellointestinal duct (connection between the midgut and the yolk sac) of the developing gut. It is present in only 2% of individuals. Look for this about 2 feet (60 cm) proximal to the ileocaecal junction in the ante-mesenteric border of the ileum. The Meckel's diverticulum may often have pancreatic or gastric mucosa as a lining, resulting in ulceration and bleeding.

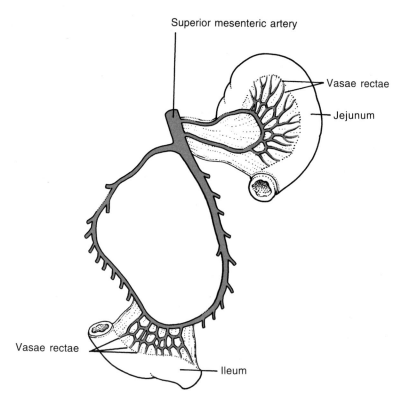

Fig. 20.3 **Jejunal and ileal arteries showing the difference in their patterns of distribution**

Large intestine

The large intestine consists of the *caecum, ascending colon, transverse colon, descending colon* and the *sigmoid colon.* The transverse and sigmoid colon each have their own mesentery (the transverse and sigmoid mesocolon) and hence are mobile. The ascending and the descending colon are retroperitoneal structures. The caecum often has peritoneum reflected on to its posterior wall forming a retrocaecal recess and hence may be mobile.

The large intestine can be distingushed from the small intestine by observing the *taenia coli* (formed by longitudinal bands of muscle), constrictions and bulges — *haustrations* — and the presence of *appendices epiploicae* which are outpouchings of peritoneum on the large intestine containing fat.

Identify the various parts of the large intestine including its hepatic and splenic flexures. Examine the caecum and the appendix and define the small mesentery of the appendix. Define the taenia coli, haustrations (Fig. 20.2) and the appendices epiploicae. Note that there are three taenia coli and they converge together at the root of the appendix at the caecum. Also note that the appendices epiploicae are more abundant in the sigmoid colon. Examine the transverse mesocolon and the sigmoid mesocolon and define their attachments.

The large intestine is supplied by the *superior* and *inferior mesenteric arteries.* The superior mesenteric artery supplies the region up to the splenic flexure and the inferior mesenteric branches supply the region beyond. The colic arteries form a series of anastomoses giving rise to the *marginal artery* which extends from the ileocolic to the colorectal junction (Fig. 20.2).

Remove the peritoneum from the surface of the transverse mesocolon, define the middle colic artery and trace it to its origin from the superior mesenteric artery (Fig. 20.2). Similarly expose the right colic and the ileocolic branches of the superior mesenteric artery. Also expose the branches of the inferior mesenteric artery supplying the descending colon and the sigmoid colon (Fig. 20.4).

The root (base) of the appendix is on the posteromedial aspect of the caecum where the three taenia coli meet, just below the ileocaecal valve. The position of the tip of the appendix is variable (Fig 20.5). In about 75 % of cases its position is retrocaecal and in about 20% it may hang down to the pelvis. The surface marking of the root of the appendix is the McBurney's point which is the junction of the lower and middle thirds of a line connecting the umbilicus to the anterior superior iliac spine.

Interior of the small intestine and the large intestine

Put two ligatures close to the duodenojejunal flexure and incise the small intestine between the ligatures. Do the same near the ileocaecal junction. Now cut the mesentery and remove the small intestine. Open the intestine and wash out its contents. Note the difference in the mucosal folds of the jejunum and ileum. In the jejunum the circular mucosal folds, which increase the surface area by about five times are more prominent and more abundant than in the ileum. If you examine the mucosa with a hand lens you may be able to see the intestinal *villi*. In the ileum, lymphoid accumulations known as the *Peyer's patches* may also be visible.

Put two ligatures at the distal part of the descending colon and remove the large intestine by incising between ligatures. Open the caecum, clean the interior and define the ileocaecal orifice, the *ileocaecal valve* and the orifice of the appendix.

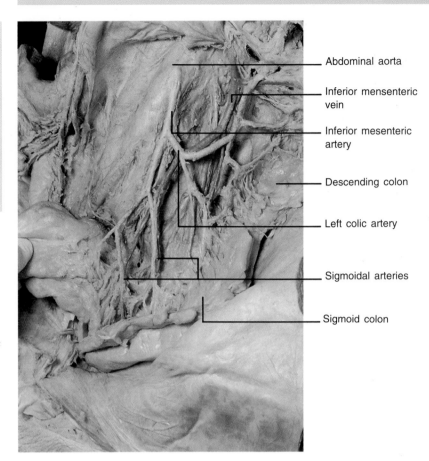

Fig. 20.4 **Inferior mesenteric artery**

- Abdominal aorta
- Inferior mensenteric vein
- Inferior mesenteric artery
- Descending colon
- Left colic artery
- Sigmoidal arteries
- Sigmoid colon

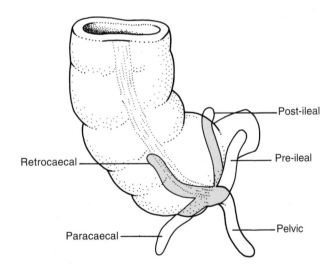

- Post-ileal
- Pre-ileal
- Retrocaecal
- Pelvic
- Paracaecal

Fig. 20.5 **The most common position of the appendix**

The coeliac trunk and coeliac plexus, duodenum, pancreas and spleen

Coeliac trunk

The coeliac trunk is the first major branch of the abdominal aorta. Its branches supply the lower part of the oesophagus, the stomach and the first half of the duodenum as well as the liver, pancreas and the spleen.

Clean the coeliac trunk in the upper part of the abdominal aorta and identify its three branches: the *common hepatic artery*, the *splenic artery* and the *left gastric artery* (Figs 21.1 & 21.2). Trace the splenic artery without damaging the accompanying splenic vein. The distribution of the left gastric and the common hepatic branches have already been examined.

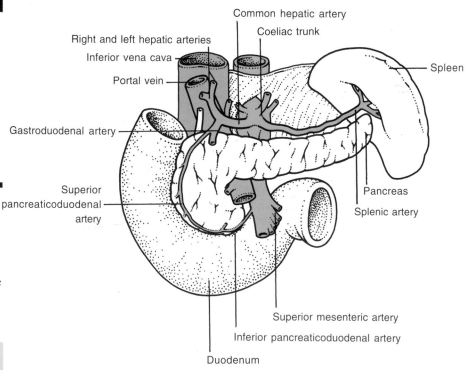

Fig. 21.1 **Common hepatic and splenic arteries**

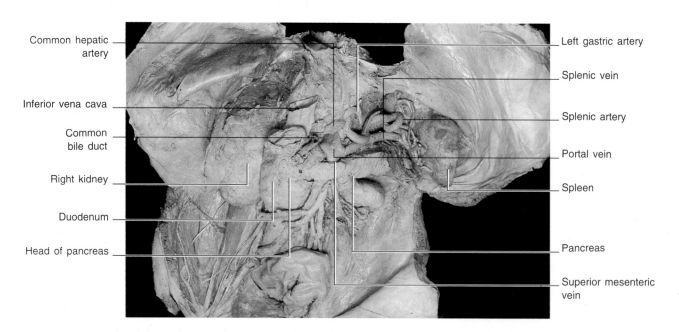

Fig. 21.2 **Duodenum, pancreas and spleen** (tail of the pancreas is removed to show the structures at the hilum of spleen)

Coeliac plexus (Fig. 21.3)

The coeliac plexus is the largest sympathetic plexus and it surrounds the coeliac trunk. The plexus receives the *greater* and *lesser splanchnic nerves* (p.44) and also a branch from the *right vagus*. The two *coeliac ganglia*, in which the preganglionic fibres of the splanchnic nerves synapse, lie on the crura of the diaphragm. Each ganglion is about 2 cm in diameter. A large contribution of preganglionic fibres from the plexus supply the adrenal medulla. The rest of the plexus descends over the abdominal aorta and is distributed to the abdominal viscera as plexuses accompanying the branches of the aorta.

Define as much of the coeliac plexus as possible. Also try to identify the coeliac ganglia. The right ganglion is overlapped by the inferior vena cava and the left by the pancreas and the splenic artery.

＊ Pain from the abdominal viscera is transmitted through the afferent sympathetic fibres in the coeliac plexus. Coeliac plexus block obtained with an anaesthetic drug is therapeutically used to relieve intractable abdominal pain — produced in conditions such as chronic pancreatitis and carcinoma of the pancreas.

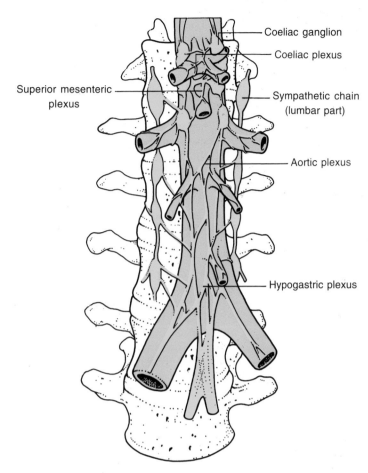

Fig. 21.3 **Prevertebral autonomic plexuses**

Duodenum (Fig. 21.1)

The duodenum is C-shaped and is divided into four parts for descriptive purposes. The head of the pancreas is surrounded by the duodenum. The first part extends upwards and to the right from the pylorus towards the liver. It is related to the liver and gallbladder anteriorly and has the gastroduodenal artery, the common bile duct and the hepatic portal vein crossing its posterior surface. The second part descends vertically downwards and is related to the hilum of the right kidney (Fig. 21.2) and the ureter. The main pancreatic duct often (80%) joins the bile duct and together they form the hepato-pancreatic *ampulla of Vater* (Fig. 21.4). The opening of the ampulla is about 8–10 cm distal to the pylorus and is guarded by the *sphincter of Oddi*. This is also the junction between the foregut and the midgut of the developing gut. The third part

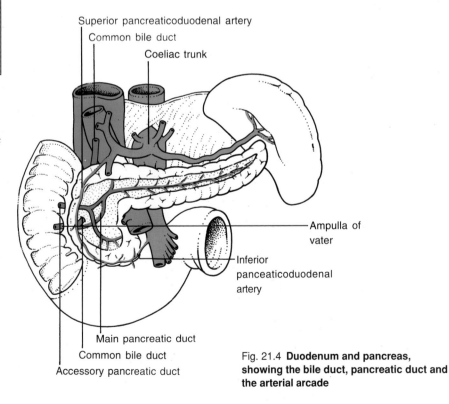

Fig. 21.4 **Duodenum and pancreas, showing the bile duct, pancreatic duct and the arterial arcade**

is horizontal and the fourth ascends vertically upwards towards the duodeno-jejunal flexure.

Verify the parts and relations of the duodenum. Trace the common bile duct through the pancreas and note its opening in the duodenum. Dissect into the pancreas and identify the termination of the pancreatic duct. Lift the duodenum from the pancreas and dissect out the *superior* and *inferior pancreatico-duodenal arteries* supplying the duodenum. Note that the inferior pancreatico-duodenal artery is a branch of the superior mesenteric artery. Trace the superior mesenteric artery to its origin from the abdominal aorta.

※ The first part of the duodenum is the site of *duodenal ulcers*. The first half of this portion of the duodenum has a peritoneal covering similar to the stomach and is mobile. Ulcers on the posterior wall of the duodenum can produce bleeding from the *gastroduodenal artery*.

Pancreas (Figs 21.1, 21.2 & 21.4)

The pancreas, lying transversely across the posterior abdominal wall, has four parts: *head*, *neck*, *body* and *tail*. The head of the pancreas is closely related to the duodenum and the common bile duct. The hepatic portal vein is formed behind the *neck* of the pancreas. The *body* of the pancreas crosses the abdominal aorta and the left kidney. The *tail* of the pancreas which is in the lienorenal ligament reaches the hilum of the spleen. The pancreas is supplied by the *splenic artery* and is drained by the *splenic vein*.

Examine the pancreas and verify its parts and relations. The shape of the pancreas may be markedly altered due to postmortem autolysis. Expose the main pancreatic duct (Fig. 21.4) as much as possible by removing the overlying pancreatic tissue. See the formation of the duct system; the interlobular ducts join the main duct almost vertically giving it a 'herring bone' appearance. Remove part of the pancreas and expose the splenic and the superior mesenteric vessels more fully.

※ As the bile duct is intimately related to the head of the pancreas, *carcinoma of the head of pancreas* blocks the bile duct and produces *obstructive jaundice*. This may be an early manifestation of the disease.

Hepatic portal vein (Fig. 21.5)

The hepatic portal vein is formed by the union of the *superior mesenteric* and the *splenic veins* behind the neck of the pancreas. The *inferior mesenteric vein* may join the splenic vein or the superior mesenteric vein. In its course towards the porta hepatis the portal vein lies behind the first part of the duodenum and in the free border of the lesser omentum.

Define the formation of the hepatic portal vein. Examine the remains of its tributaries.

※ The portal vein tributaries anastomose with those of the systemic veins forming *porto-systemic anastomoses* (Fig. 21.5). In *portal hypertension* the anastomosis at the lower end of the oesophagus enlarges and produce *oesophageal varices* which can suddenly rupture, resulting in severe *haematemesis* (vomiting of blood) which can be fatal.

Spleen

The spleen has *diaphragmatic* and *visceral* surfaces. The diaphragm separates the spleen from ribs 9–11 as well as the left lung and pleura. The visceral surface is related to the stomach, the splenic flexure of the colon and the left kidney. The hilum of the spleen is related to the tail of the pancreas, the splenic vessels and lymph nodes. The spleen is almost completely invested by peritoneum and is connected to the stomach and the left kidney by gastrosplenic and lienorenal ligaments respectively.

Examine the spleen and its relations. Dissect the hilum of the spleen and verify the relation to the left kidney. Note that the spleen has prominent notches on its anterior border.

※ The spleen may be enlarged in many conditions. It is sometimes difficult to distinguish it from an enlarged left kidney. Feeling the splenic notches verifies the identification of spleen. Spleen has to enlarge to at least twice its normal size before it can be felt.

※ Although the spleen is protected under the costal margin, it is more prone to rupture than any other abdominal organ. A normal spleen can rupture due to a severe blow on the abdomen or on lower thorax on the left side. An enlarged and diseased spleen can rupture spontaneously or after trivial trauma. Rupture of spleen causes bleeding into the peritoneal cavity, resulting in shock.

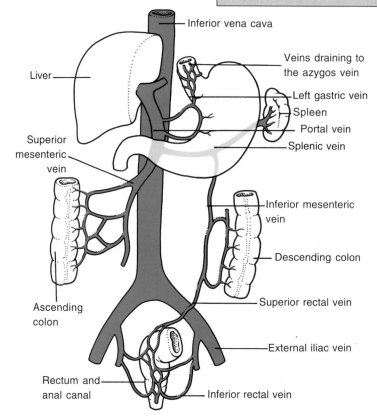

Fig. 21.5 **Formation of the portal vein and the portosystemic anastomoses**

22

The kidneys, adrenal glands, diaphragm and the posterior abdominal wall

This dissection will examine the kidneys, the adrenal glands, the aorta, and the inferior vena cava as well as the diaphragm and the posterior abdominal wall.

Remove the duodenum, pancreas and spleen. Expose the kidneys and the adrenal glands by removing their fat and fascial coverings. Clean the *renal artery*, the *renal vein* and the *ureter* at the *hilum* of the kidney on both sides (Fig. 22.1). At the hilum the vein lies in front, the ureter at the back and the artery in between. Often the renal artery may branch outside the kidney and there may be more than one artery entering the kidney.

Note that the left renal vein crosses in front of the aorta to reach the inferior vena cava.

Kidney

The kidney is covered by *renal fascia* and the *perirenal fat*. These coverings along with the renal vessels anchor the kidney on the posterior abdominal wall. The hilum of the kidney is in the transpyloric plane about 5 cm from the midline, its upper pole lies 2.5 cm and the lower pole 7.5 cm away from the midline. Posteriorly, the kidneys lie on the diaphragm, the psoas major, the quadratus lumborum and the transversus abdominis (Fig. 22.2). Their anterior relations are shown in Figure 22.3.

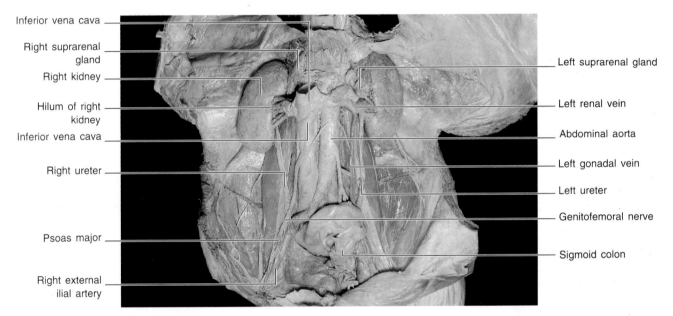

Fig. 22.1 **Structures on the posterior abdominal wall**

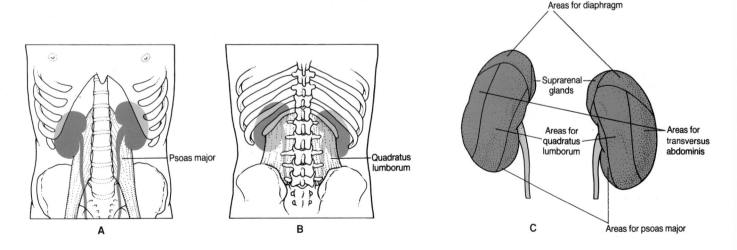

Fig. 22.2 **Posterior relations of the kidney. A.** Anterior view. **B.** Posterior view. **C.** Areas marked on the posterior surfaces of the kidneys

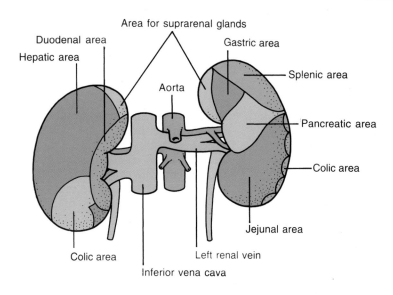

Fig. 22.3 **Anterior surfaces of the kidneys**

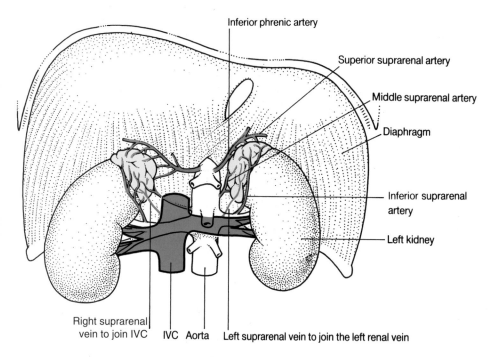

Fig. 22.4 **Kidneys and suprarenal glands: anterior view**

Clean the *ureters*. Note that they lie on the psoas major muscles which separate the ureters from the transverse processes of the vertebrae. The ureter enters the pelvis by crossing superficial to the termination of the common iliac artery. The course of the pelvic part of the ureter will be examined later.

Adrenal glands

Examine the adrenal glands. Make an attempt to dissect out their blood supply (Fig. 22.4).

The adrenal (suprarenal) glands lie on the upper poles of the kidneys. The right gland lies behind the liver and the inferior vena cava and the left behind the stomach and the pancreas. Each gland is supplied by three arteries and drained by one vein.

Incise the renal arteries and the renal veins. Cut the ureters in the lower part of the abdomen. Remove the kidneys and the adrenal glands. Examine the structures at the hilum of the kidney and note their positions. Slice the kidney longitudinally and examine the cut surface (Fig. 22.5). Identify the *cortex, medulla,* and the *major and minor calyces* as well as the *pelvis of the ureter.*

Clean the *inferior vena cava* and the *abdominal aorta.* Identify the cut ends of the branches of the aorta. Define the *gonadal artery* (testicular artery in the male and ovarian artery in the female), one on each side. Dissect the *lumbar arteries* (usually four in number) branching off from the sides of the aorta and the accompanying *lumbar veins.* Look for the *median sacral artery* arising from the bifurcation of the aorta.

The aorta terminates by dividing into the right and left *common iliac arteries.* Each common iliac artery divides to form the *external* and *internal iliac arteries.* These arteries are accompanied by the corresponding veins. The two *common iliac veins* join to form the *inferior vena cava.*

The *surface marking of the aorta* extends from a point just above the transpyloric plane in the midline to a point just to the left of the midline in a plane connecting the highest points of the iliac crests. The common iliac and the external iliac arteries can be marked by extending the line on either side to a point midway between the anterior superior iliac spine and the pubic symphysis.

Posterior abdominal wall

Incise the upper part of the aorta and the inferior vena cava and remove them. Clean the muscles of the posterior abdominal wall (Fig. 22.6). Define the *subcostal, iliohypogastric* and *lateral cutaneous nerves of the thigh* emerging from the lateral border of the psoas major muscle. Identify the genitofemoral nerve on the anterior surface of the psoas. Define the *lumbar sympathetic trunk* along the medial border of the psoas (Fig. 22.6).

The lumbar part of the sympathetic chain lies along the anterolateral surface of the bodies of the lumbar vertebrae and along the medial border of the psoas. There are usually four ganglia in the lumbar region. The left lumbar sympathetic chain is overlapped by the aorta and the right by the inferior vena cava. Postganglionic fibres from the lumbar ganglia (*grey rami*) are distributed to the lumbar spinal nerves. The *lumbar splanchnic nerves* are preganglionic fibres connecting the ganglia to the aortic plexus (See Fig. 21.3 p.75).

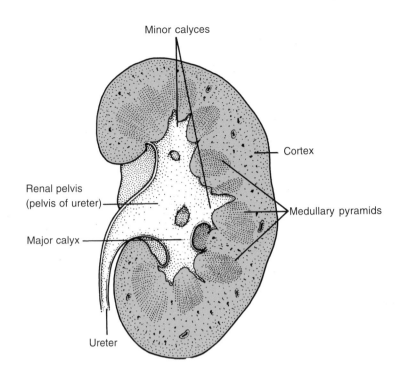

Fig. 22.5 **Cut surface of the kidney**

✳ *Lumbar sympathectomy.* This is undertaken surgically or by producing neurolysis by injection of chemical agents such as phenol or alcohol. The procedure interrupts vasoconstrictor fibres and is undertaken in cases of peripheral vascular disease of the lower limb.

Verify the attachment of the psoas major to the vertebral bodies and the transverse processes. Define and clean the quadratus lumborum muscle which lies lateral to the psoas major.

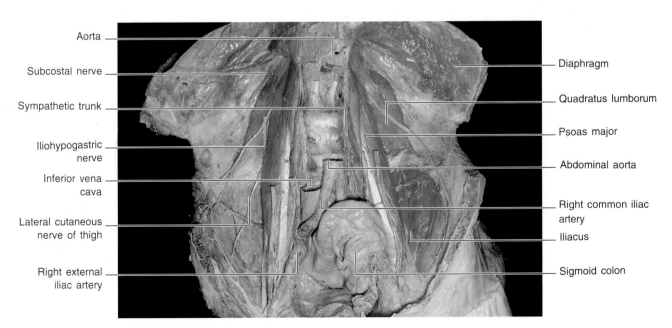

Fig. 22.6 **Muscles of the posterior abdominal wall**

Diaphragm

The diaphragm is a dome shaped muscle separating the thoracic from the abdominal cavity. Its entire motor innervation is derived from the *phrenic nerves* (C3,4,5). It transmits the inferior vena cava, the oesophagus, the sympathetic trunk and the splanchnic nerves. The aorta passes behind the diaphragm. The peripheral part of the diaphragm is muscular where as its central part, the *central tendon*, is fibrous. The muscular part is attached to the upper lumbar vertebrae and the intervertebral discs through the right and left *crura*. The aorta passes between the two crura, hence is behind the diaphragm. Fibres of the diaphragm also take origin from the medial and lateral *arcuate ligaments* which are thickenings of the fascia overlying the psoas major and the quadratus lumborum muscles on the posterior abdominal wall (Fig 22.7). Besides the vertebral attachments the diaphragm is also attached to the inner aspects of the lower six ribs and costal cartilages as well as to the xiphoid process of the sternum.

Examine the diaphragm (Fig. 22.7). Define its attachments to the vertebrae through the crura and the medial and lateral *arcuate ligaments*. Note the aortic opening in between the two crura.

The *aortic opening* lies at the level of T12. The *oesophagus* passes through the left crus with the fibres of the right crus looping around it at the level of T10. The *inferior vena caval opening*, at the level of T8, lies more anteriorly in the central tendon of the diaphragm. The *sympathetic trunk* enters the abdomen by passing under the medial arcuate ligament, and the *splanchnic nerves* by piercing the crura.

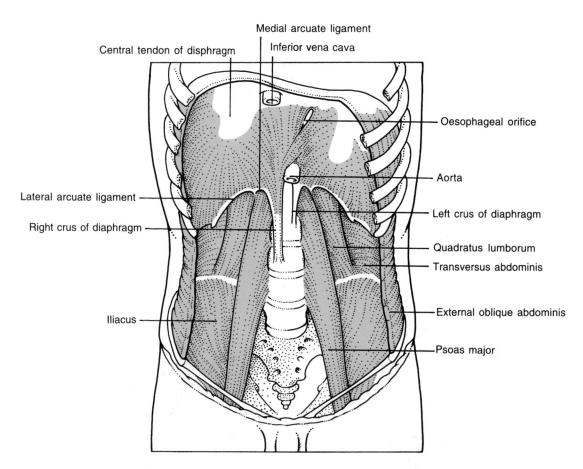

Central tendon of disphragm

Medial arcuate ligament

Inferior vena cava

Oesophageal orifice

Aorta

Lateral arcuate ligament

Left crus of diaphragm

Right crus of diaphragm

Quadratus lumborum

Transversus abdominis

External oblique abdominis

Iliacus

Psoas major

Fig. 22.7 **Muscles of the posterior abdominal wall and the diaphragm: anterior view**

23

The pelvis

The pelvis contains the terminal parts of the alimentary and urinary systems and also parts of the reproductive system. In this session these organs will be examined in situ before they are removed for further examination during the next session.

OSTEOLOGY

The bony pelvis (Fig. 23.1) is made up of three bones: the two *hip bones* and the *sacrum*. The hip bones articulate with each other in front at the pubic symphysis and with the sacrum at the back through the two sacroiliac joints. Each hip bone has three components, viz. the *ilium*, the *pubis* and the *ischium*, which fuse together in the acetabulum.

Refer to Figure 23.1 and identify the main features of the bony pelvis.

The cavity of the pelvis contains the *rectum* and the *urinary bladder*. In the female it contains the *uterus* and the upper part of the *vagina*. These organs are supported and their normal positions are maintained by a sheet of muscle in the lower part of the pelvis. The muscle is the *pelvic diaphragm* and is mostly formed by the two *levator ani* muscles which fuse in the midline.

Examine the general relations of the pelvic organs in both male and female.

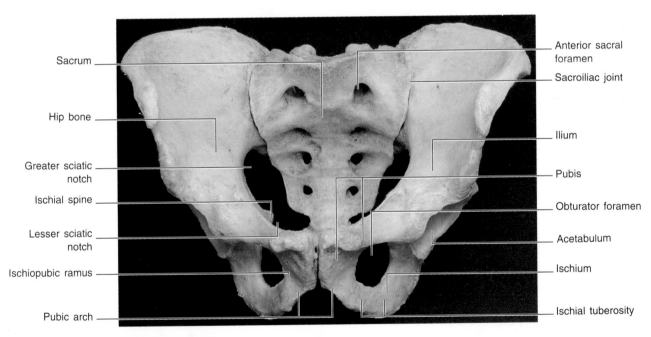

Fig. 23.1 **Bony pelvis**

Female

Examine the female pelvis. Refer to Figure 23.2 and identify the uterus with the urinary bladder in front and the rectum behind. (*Hysterectomy* — removal of the uterus — is a common operation and hence this organ may be missing in your specimen.)

Notice how the sigmoid colon becomes the rectum and also note the differences between the two.

The *sigmoid colon* has a mesentery, the *sigmoid mesocolon*, whereas there is no peritoneum behind the rectum. The rectum is more fixed than the sigmoid colon. The taenia coli and the appendices epiploicae seen in the sigmoid colon are absent in the rectum.

Peritoneum

At the junction between the lower and the middle third of the rectum, the peritoneum is reflected forward onto the posterior surface of the vagina. The peritoneal space thus formed between the rectum and the uterus and vagina is the most dependent part of the peritoneal cavity and is known as the *recto-uterine pouch*.

Pull the uterus forward and examine the recto-uterine pouch. Note that anteriorly the peritoneum from the bladder is reflected onto the superior surface of the urinary bladder forming the *uterovesical pouch* in between the bladder and the uterus (Fig. 23.2). Define the *broad ligament*

which is a double-layered peritoneal membrane extending laterally from the uterus. Feel the *uterine tube* along the upper border of the broad ligament. The lateral end of the uterine tube has the fimbriae. Identify the *ovary* next to the fimbriae. The ovary is connected to the broad ligament by the *mesovarium*.

Trace the *pelvic part of the ureter* in the female and note its relations to the common iliac artery and the branches of the internal iliac arteries (Fig. 23.5). Verify that the *uterine artery* is crossing above the ureter close to the *lateral fornix of the vagina*.

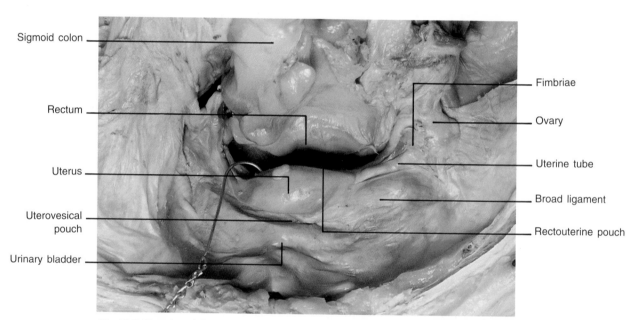

Sigmoid colon

Rectum

Uterus

Uterovesical pouch

Urinary bladder

Fimbriae

Ovary

Uterine tube

Broad ligament

Rectouterine pouch

Fig. 23.2 **Female pelvis seen from above**

✳ During *hysterectomy*, while the surgeon ligates and cuts the uterine arteries, the ureters are in danger of being clamped or cut inadvertently.

Male

Refer to Figure 23.3 and identify the *urinary bladder* and the *rectum* and the peritoneal space between the two, the *rectovesical pouch*. The rectovesical pouch is the most dependent part of the peritoneal cavity in the male. Palpate the *seminal vesicle* and the *ductus deferens* behind the bladder. Study the rectum and the sigmoid colon as in the female.

Remove the peritoneum covering the rectum and the bladder. Note that the peritoneal relations of these organs are similar to those in the female and that only the superior surface of the bladder is covered by peritoneum.

Refer to Figure 23.4 and trace the *ureter* towards the bladder by removing the peritoneum. Note that it enters the pelvis by crossing in front of the bifurcation of the *common iliac artery*. It then lies on the side wall of the pelvis where it is related to the *obturator nerve*, *obturator artery* and other branches of the *internal iliac artery*. Trace the ductus deferens and note that it crosses the ureter before reaching the posterior surface of the bladder.

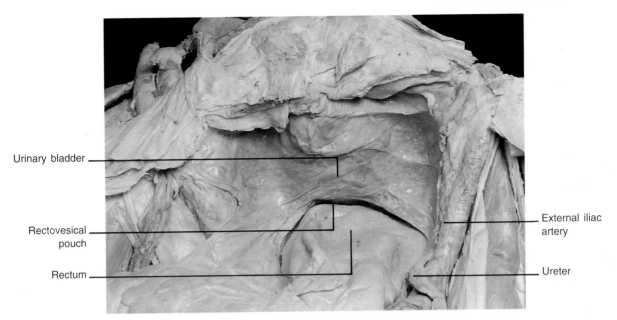

Urinary bladder

Rectovesical pouch

Rectum

External iliac artery

Ureter

Fig. 23.3 **Male pelvis seen from above**

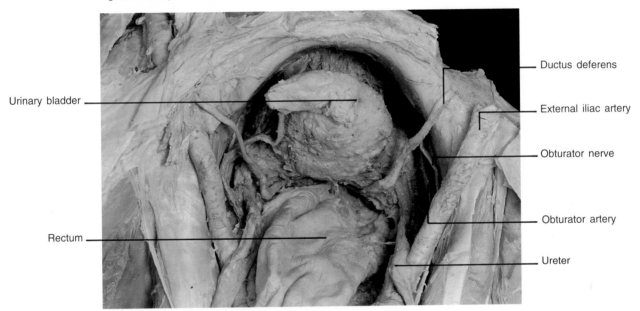

Urinary bladder

Rectum

Ductus deferens

External iliac artery

Obturator nerve

Obturator artery

Ureter

Fig. 23.4 **Course of the pelvic part of the ureter in the male**

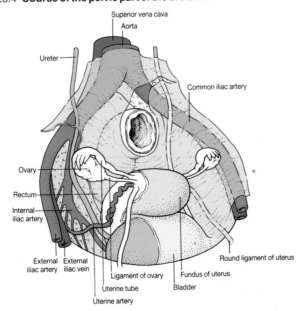

Superior vena cava

Aorta

Ureter

Common iliac artery

Ovary

Rectum

Internal iliac artery

External iliac artery

External iliac vein

Uterine tube

Uterine artery

Ligament of ovary

Bladder

Fundus of uterus

Round ligament of uterus

Fig. 23.5 **Female pelvic organs seen from above (diagrammatic).** The peritoneum on the right side has been partially removed

24

The male pelvic organs

During this session the pelvic organs in the male will be examined. For better visualization some of the organs may have to be removed before their detailed structure is examined.

Note again the difference between the rectum and the sigmoid colon. Remove the peritoneum from the front of the rectum. Note that anteriorly the rectum is related to the back of the bladder, the seminal vesicles and the ductus deferens. Posteriorly it is related to the sacrum, sacral plexus and the piriformis muscle (p.82).

The condensed pelvic fascia behind the rectum is the *Waldeyer's fascia* and it contains the plexus of veins draining the rectum. The rectum follows the curvature of the sacrum and also has three lateral flexures. The lower part of the rectum is expanded to form the *ampulla of the rectum*.

Refer to Figure 24.1 and clean the *superior rectal artery* supplying the rectum. This is a continuation of the inferior mesenteric artery and it supplies the rectum and the upper part of the anal canal. The *middle rectal artery* is small and is a branch of the internal iliac artery. The *inferior rectal artery* supplies the anal canal and anastomoses with the superior rectal artery.

Insert your finger below the bladder and feel the prostate gland. Make an incision below the prostate and remove the prostate, bladder, seminal vesicles, ductus deferens and ureters in one piece. To do this incise the ureters and the ductus deferens as they enter the pelvis and also cut the superior and inferior vesical arteries from the internal iliac artery as they enter the bladder. Examine the bladder.

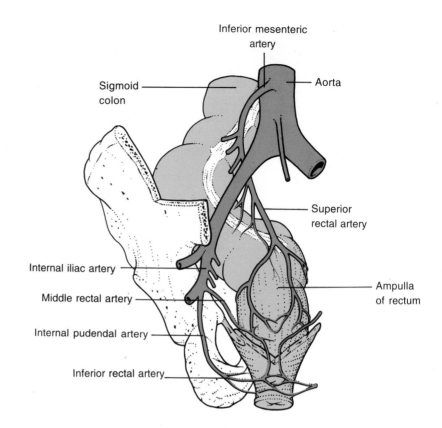

Fig. 24.1 **Arterial supply of the rectum and anal canal — posterior view**

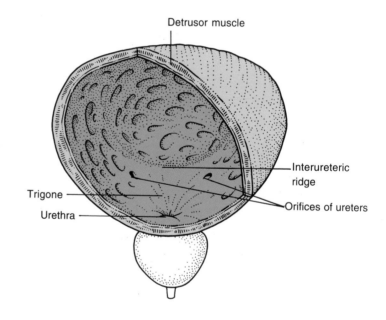

Fig. 24.2 **Inside of the bladder**

The urinary bladder

The empty bladder has a superior surface, two inferolateral surfaces and a base. The base faces posteriorly. The lower part of the bladder which is continuous with the urethra is known as the *bladder neck*. Only the superior surface is covered by peritoneum.

Incise the bladder from the front and examine the inside. The mucosa of the empty bladder is thrown into folds; these flatten as the bladder distends. The inner aspect of the posterior wall however is smooth. This is known as the *trigone of the bladder* and is bounded laterally by the opening of the two ureters and below by the urethra (Fig. 24.2). In the upper border of the trigone is the *interureteric ridge* (interureteric bar) which extends between the two ureteric orifices. The interureteric ridge can be seen during *cystoscopy* (examination of the interior of the bladder). The two ureters will be seen discharging urine at its two ends. The ureters lie obliquely in the bladder wall before their termination and have a valve-like mechanism which prevents reflux of urine into them during contraction of the bladder.

The mucosa of the bladder is lined by *transitional epithelium* which will not absorb urine. Remove the mucosa and examine the underlying muscle. This is the *detrusor muscle* the fibres of which run in different directions and interlace with each other.

* In *urinary obstruction* the detrusor muscle hypertrophies and the spaces in between the muscle fibres deepen to give rise to bladder diverticulae. Urine will collect in the diverticulae without draining and predispose to infection of the bladder.

The muscle of the trigone is different from the detrusor. It extends into the lower part of the ureters and also into the urethra. At the bladder neck the trigonal muscle is circular in the male and forms the *internal sphincter of the bladder*. This prevents regurgitation of semen into the bladder during ejaculation.

The bladder is innervated by sympathetic and parasympathetic nerves. The motor supply to the detrusor is from the parasympathetic (*pelvic splanchnic nerves*) and that to the trigonal muscle and the internal sphincter is by the sympathetic. Pain from the bladder is transmitted by both sets of nerves.

Examine the ductus deferens and the seminal vesicles lying behind the bladder (Fig. 24.3). Note that the ductus deferens lies medial to the seminal vesicles.

The *ductus deferens (vas deferens)* starts at the inferior pole of the testis as a continuation of the epididymis. It passes through the inguinal canal and the deep inguinal ring before reaching the posterior surface of the bladder. The dilatation just before its termination is the *ampulla of the vas deferens*. The ductus terminates by joining the duct of the seminal vesicle to form the *ejaculatory duct*.

* The *seminal vesicles* secrete the bulk of the seminal fluid. Rarely, the seminal vesicle may become infected and then tenderness may be felt during rectal examination. Normal seminal vesicles are not palpable per rectum.

Examine the *prostate gland*. Note that the urethra and the two ejaculatory ducts pass through the prostate. The ejaculatory ducts drain into the *prostatic part of the urethra*.

The posterior surface of the prostate has a groove which is normally felt on *rectal examination*. When the prostate enlarges this groove disappears. Veins of the prostate drain into the *prostatic venous plexus* around the gland. This in turn is connected to the *vertebral venous plexuses* (Batson's veins). There are no valves in these connections.

* Malignant tumours of the prostate spread through these veins into the vertebral column.

The prostate contains fibro-muscular tissue and glands which open into the urethra. Prostatic secretion adds to the seminal fluid.

* Benign tumours of the prostate are extremely common in men above the age of 60. It is the *median lobe of the prostate* which is usually affected by benign hypertrophy. The median lobe is bounded by the two ejaculatory ducts and the urethra and contains small glands which are not coiled. The rest of the prostatic tissue is divided into *posterior, lateral* and *anterior lobes* (Fig. 24.4). Glands of the lateral and posterior lobes are long and tortuous and are affected by malignant growths.

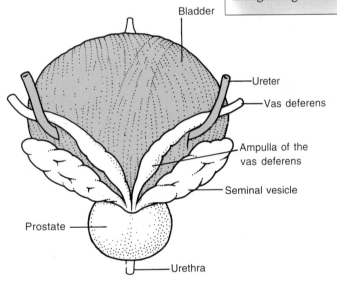

Fig. 24.3 **Posterior surface of the bladder in the male**

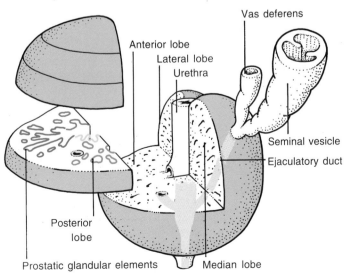

Fig. 24.4 **Lobes of the prostate and the ejaculatory duct**

25

The female pelvic organs

Those who are dissecting female cadavers will examine the pelvic organs in the female during this session.

Examination of the rectum and its blood supply should be conducted as described for the male (p.84). Note that in the female, the rectum is related anteriorly to the vagina, the uterus and the recto-uterine pouch.

Incise the vagina as close to the pelvic diaphragm as possible and remove the urinary bladder, the upper part of the vagina, uterus, broad ligament, uterine tube and the ovaries en masse. You will have to sever the blood vessels of these organs as you do this.

Urinary bladder

Study the *urinary bladder*. Posteriorly it is related to the uterus. Examine the interior of the bladder as described for the male (p.84). Identify the *trigone* and the *interureteric ridge*. The muscle fibres in the trigone continue into the urethra. However, unlike in the male urinary bladder, these fibres are longitudinal in direction and hence do not form a sphincter at the *bladder neck*.

Ovaries

Examine the *ovaries*. Each ovary is ovoid in shape and is attached to the posterior leaf of the *broad ligament* by a double fold of peritoneum, the *mesovarium*. Continuation of the broad ligament from the ovary to the side wall of the pelvis is known as the *suspensory ligament of the ovary* (Fig. 25.1).

The ovary lies on the side wall of the pelvis in the 'ovarian fossa', in the angle between the external and internal iliac vessels. The ureter lies close behind the ovary.

The ovary in its normal position may be just palpable by *vaginal examination*. It is laterally related to the *obturator nerve*.

✳ Inflammation of the ovary may cause pain along the distribution of the obturator nerve, along the medial aspect of the thigh.

Examine the side wall of the pelvis and identify the ovarian fossa and the obturator nerve.

Peel off the peritoneum covering the ovary and define the *ligament of the ovary* connecting it to the uterus. This ligament then extends to the labium majus through the inguinal canal as the round ligament of the uterus.

The ovary is supplied by the *ovarian artery* given off just below the renal artery from the abdominal aorta. Veins form a plexus which eventually form a single trunk. On the left side this drains into the left renal vein and on the right side into the inferior vena cava. The lymphatics of the ovary drain into the para-aortic nodes. The blood supply of the ovaries and their lymphatic drainage are comparable to those of the testes (p.63).

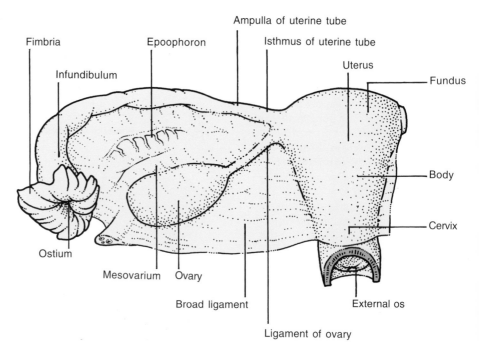

Fig. 25.1 **Uterus, broad ligament and ovary: posterior view**

Uterus

Study the *uterus*. Identify the *funaus*, *body* and *cervix* of the uterus. Note that the lower part of the cervix is inside the vagina (Fig. 25.1).

The spaces around the cervix, inside the vagina, are the vaginal fornices. They are divided into anterior, posterior and lateral fornices according to their positions in relation to the vagina. The posterior fornix is deeper than the others. The opening of the cervix into the vagina is the *external os*.

In its normal position the uterus is angulated forward on the vagina (Fig. 25.2). This is known as the *anteverted* position of the uterus and it is maintained by the levator ani (pelvic diaphragm) and the various ligaments connected to the uterus and vagina (Fig. 26.2 p.88).

Peritoneum covers the whole of the posterior surface and upper third of the vagina and is reflected onto the rectum forming the recto-uterine pouch.

✳ Anteriorly, the supravaginal part of the cervix is not covered by peritoneum. This part enlarges during pregnancy and becomes the *lower segment of the uterus;* this is the usual site of caesarean sections.

Remove the peritoneum from the surface of the uterus and trace the *uterine artery* upwards on the lateral aspect of the uterus. The artery crosses above the ureter, adjacent to the lateral fornix (p.82), before ascending up in the broad ligament on the side of the uterus. Also trace the ovarian artery along the uterine tube and note the anastomoses between the uterine and the ovarian arteries (Fig. 25.3).

Examine the *uterine tube*. It ends laterally by opening near the ovary. The opening is called the *osteum*. The tube lies inside the broad ligament. The osteum allows the tube to communicate with the peritoneal cavity.

Refer to Figure 25.1 and identify the *infundibulum, ampulla, isthmus* and *intramural parts of the uterine tub*e.

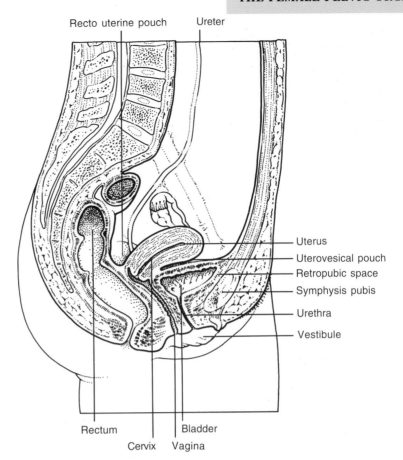

Fig. 25.2 **Female pelvis: sagittal section**

Labels: Recto uterine pouch, Ureter, Uterus, Uterovesical pouch, Retropubic space, Symphysis pubis, Urethra, Vestibule, Rectum, Bladder, Cervix, Vagina

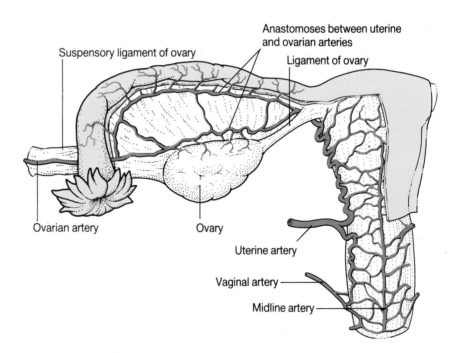

Fig. 25.3 **Arterial supply of the ovary, uterine tube, uterus and vagina**

Labels: Suspensory ligament of ovary, Anastomoses between uterine and ovarian arteries, Ligament of ovary, Ovarian artery, Ovary, Uterine artery, Vaginal artery, Midline artery

✳ The patency of the tube is essential for normal pregnancy. Infection of the tube (*salpingitis*) may result in scarring and closure of the tubes. In *tubal sterilizatio*n the uterine tubes are cut to prevent future pregnancies. In tubal *ectopic pregnancies* the fertilized ovum may implant in the uterine tube instead of passing into the uterus. However, the tube cannot accommodate the growing fetus and the placenta, and will rupture into the peritoneal cavity resulting in bleeding and peritonitis.

26

The pelvic wall

In this session the structures on the pelvic wall will be examined.

Refer to Figure 23.1 (p.81) and revise the osteology of the bony pelvis.

Three pairs of muscles are seen on the walls of the pelvis. The side wall has the *obturator internus* muscle covering the obturator foramen. Posteriorly, taking origin from the sacrum and passing through the greater sciatic foramen is the *piriformis muscle*. The two *levator ani* form the floor of the pelvis.

Refer to Figure 26.1 and clean the levator ani, obturator internus and the piriformis. Note that the two levator ani muscles fuse in the midline to form a gutter.

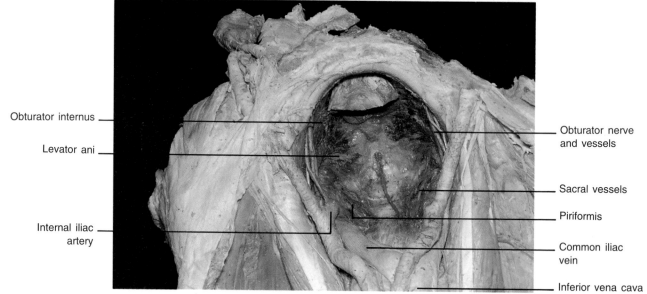

Obturator internus

Levator ani

Internal iliac artery

Obturator nerve and vessels

Sacral vessels

Piriformis

Common iliac vein

Inferior vena cava

Fig. 26.1 **Muscles of the pelvis seen from above**

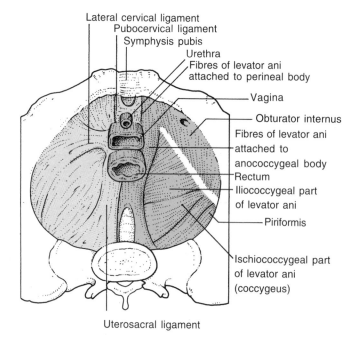

Lateral cervical ligament
Pubocervical ligament
Symphysis pubis
Urethra
Fibres of levator ani attached to perineal body

Vagina

Obturator internus
Fibres of levator ani attached to anococcygeal body
Rectum
Iliococcygeal part of levator ani

Piriformis

Ischiococcygeal part of levator ani (coccygeus)

Uterosacral ligament

Fig. 26.2 **Floor of the pelvis and muscles and ligaments supporting the uterus and vagina: superior view.** Ligaments are shown on the left side and muscles on the right

The *levator ani* takes origin from a line extending from the back of the pubis to the ischial spine and is described as having three parts: the *pubococcygeus*, the *iliococcygeus* and the *ischiococcygeus* (Fig. 26.2). The iliococcygeus does not arise from the ilium but instead is attached to the fascia covering the obturator internus muscle.

The fibres of the levator ani run downwards, medially and backwards. As they do so, the inner fibres of pubococcygeus are intimately related to the pelvic organs. The muscle is important in maintaining the normal positions of the pelvic organs. Fibres of the levator ani related to the prostate are known as the *levator prostatae*; those around the vagina form the *sphincter vaginae*. Behind these the fibres are inserted into a tough fibromuscular nodule, the *perineal body*, in front of the anorectal junction. A number of perineal muscles are also inserted into the perineal body (Fig. 27.5, p.93). The perineal body together with the muscles attached to it prevent the pelvic organs from prolapsing into the perineum.

The part of the levator ani around the anorectal junction is called the *puborectalis muscle*. The puborectalis fibres form a sling around the anorectal junction, i.e. fibres of one side become continuous with those of the opposite side. This sling maintains the forward angulation of the anorectal junction. Fibres of the sling also fuse with the deep part of the external sphincter of the anal canal and contribute to the formation of the *anorectal ring*. This forms an important part of the sphincteric mechanism in the anorectal region.

The more lateral fibres of the levator ani fuse in a fibrous raphe behind the anorectal junction, the *anococcygeal raphe*.

Examine the piriformis. This takes origin from the sacrum and leaves through the greater sciatic foramen to be inserted into the greater trochanter of the femur. The piriformis, as well as the obturator internus muscle are described in the section on the gluteal region of the lower limb (p.109).

The components of the *sacral plexus* are also seen on the posterior wall of the pelvis (Fig. 26.3).

> Clean the ventral rami of the sacral nerves emerging through the anterior sacral foramina. Identify the lumbosacral trunk crossing the pelvic brim and contributing to the sacral plexus.

Most of the nerves formed in the sacral plexus leave the pelvis through the greater sciatic foramen. They will be further examined during the dissection of the lower limb.

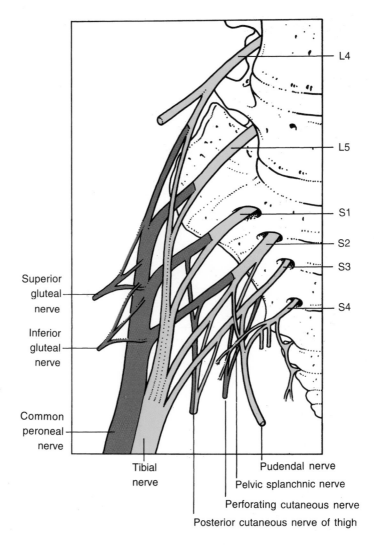

Fig. 26.3 **Sacral plexus.** The anterior division is shown in orange, the posterior division in brown

Finally clean the external and internal iliac arteries on the lateral wall of the pelvis. Also clean the obturator nerve. Branches of the internal iliac artery are shown in Figures 26.4 A&B. The visceral branches have already been cut. However, you should be able to clean the parietal branches as well as identify the cut ends of the visceral branches. Note that the *internal pudendal artery* leaves the pelvis through the greater sciatic foramen and enters the perineum through the lesser sciatic foramen. The artery accompanied by the *pudendal nerve* thus enters the perineum from the pelvis without piercing the pelvic diaphragm.

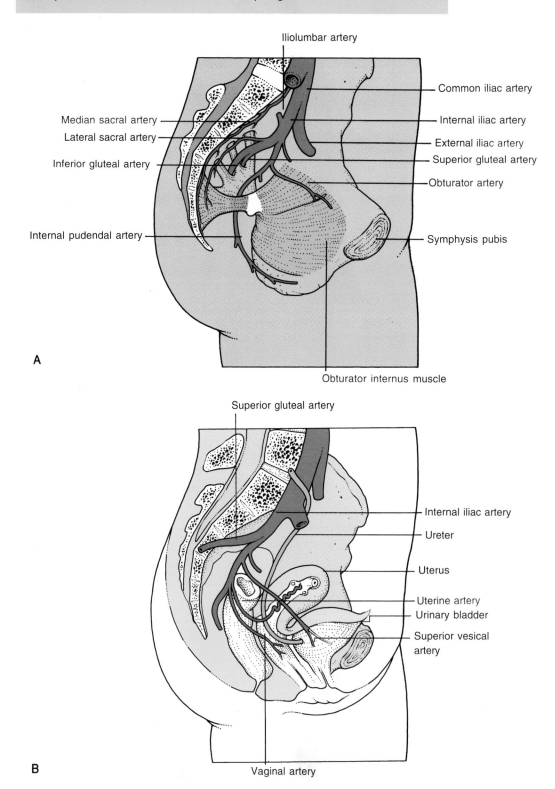

Fig. 26.4 **A. Arteries of the pelvic wall. B. Visceral branches of the internal iliac artery**

27

The perineum

The perineum is the region containing the external genitalia and the anal canal. Dissection is difficult as a number of structures are packed into this small area. Dissectors are advised to read the description before attempting to dissect this region.

Boundaries

The space below the pelvic diaphragm is defined as the perineum. The *rectum* passes through the pelvic diaphragm to become the *anal canal* in the perineum. Similarly, the vagina and the urethra also pass through the pelvic diaphragm into the perineum.

The perineum is bounded in front, behind, and laterally by the outlet of the pelvis (Fig. 27.1) and above by the pelvic diaphragm formed by the two levator ani muscles. For descriptive purposes the perineum is divided by an imaginary line connecting the two ischial tuberosities into the *anal triangle*, which contains the anal canal, and the *urogenital triangle*, containing the urethra and the external genitalia. The external aspect of the perineum has the external genitalia towards its anterior aspect and the *anus*, or the opening of the anal canal, posteriorly (Fig. 27.2).

Anal triangle

The anal triangle has the anal canal in the middle and the two *ischiorectal fossae* on either side. The ischiorectal fossa is a fat-containing space which allows expansion of the anal canal.

✳ The ischiorectal fossa can become infected and form an ischiorectal abscess which may need surgical intervention.

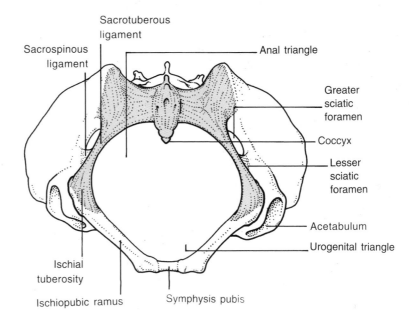

Fig. 27.1 **Boundaries of the perineum**

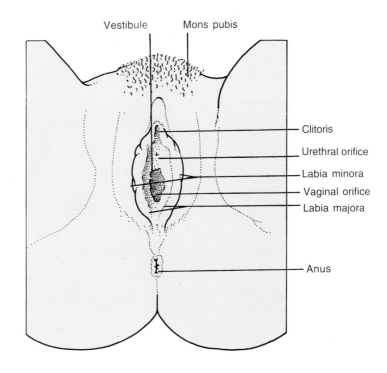

Fig. 27.2 **Female perineum showing the external genitalia**

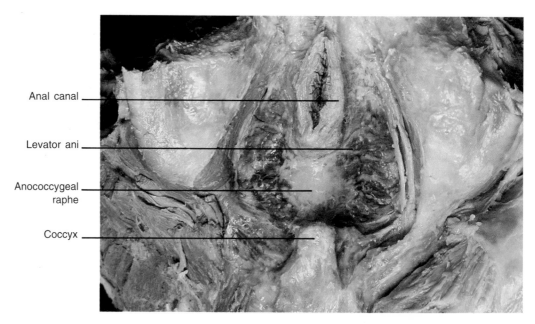

Anal canal

Levator ani

Anococcygeal raphe

Coccyx

Fig. 27.3 **Anal canal and the ischiorectal fossae.** The anococcygeal body has been removed to show the connection between the two fossae (see text)

Refer to Figures 27.3 and 27.4 and note the boundaries of the ischiorectal fossa. It is a wedge-shaped space bounded laterally by the *obturator internus* muscle and medially by the levator ani and the anal canal. The *anal canal* here is surrounded by its *external sphincter*. The obturator internus takes origin from the inner aspect of the obturator membrane covering the obturator foramen. The two ischiorectal fossae are separated in the midline, behind the anal canal, by a fibromuscular partition, the anococcygeal body. This has an opening in its upper portion through which the two ischiorectal fossae communicate with each other.

Remove the skin and the superficial fascia from the anal triangle. Using scalpel and forceps remove the fat on either side of the anal canal and expose the ischiorectal fossa. Insert your finger into the fossa and feel the boundaries of the fossa (Fig. 27.3).

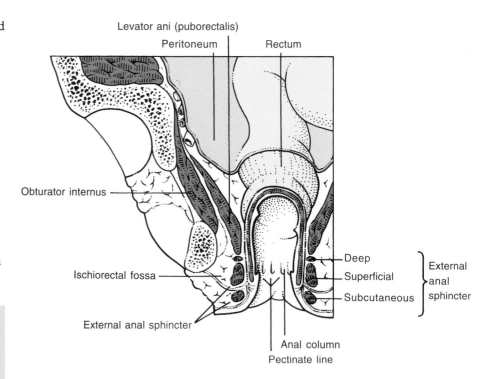

Levator ani (puborectalis)

Peritoneum

Rectum

Obturator internus

Ischiorectal fossa

External anal sphincter

Deep
Superficial
Subcutaneous

External anal sphincter

Anal column
Pectinate line

Fig. 27.4 **Section through the pelvis showing the boundaries of the ischiorectal fossa**

Urogenital triangle

As the name implies, the urogenital triangle contains parts of the reproductive system and the urethra. This part of the perineum is divided for descriptive purposes into the *superficial perineal pouch* and the *deep perineal pouch*. The partition between the two is the *perineal membrane*, a triangular sheet of fibrous tissue extending between the two ischiopubic rami (Fig. 27.5).

Superficial perineal pouch

This space is superficial to the perineal membrane and is bounded externally by the *membranous layer of the superficial fascia (Colles' fascia)*, which is an extension of the fascia from the anterior abdominal wall into the perineum. Hence, the superficial perineal pouch is continuous with the space under the membranous layer of the superficial fascia in the anterior abdominal wall.

In the male, the superficial perineal pouch contains the erectile tissues contributing to the formation of the penis and the thin muscles covering them. These are illustrated in Figure 27.6. The *urethra* passes through the corpus spongiosum of the penis.

✳ If the urethra is ruptured urine will accumulate in the superficial pouch and spread upwards into the anterior abdominal wall into which the space extends.

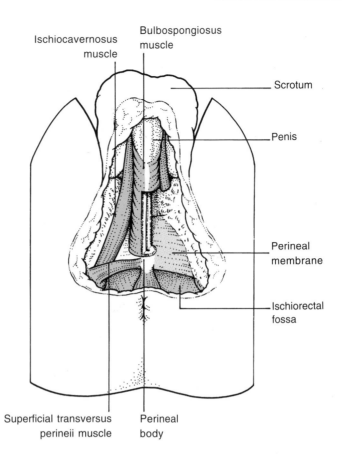

Fig. 27.5 **Muscles of the male perineum and the perineal membrane: inferior view.** The superficial muscles and part of the penis have been removed on the left-hand side of the perineum to show the perineal membrane (scrotum and the penis are lifted up)

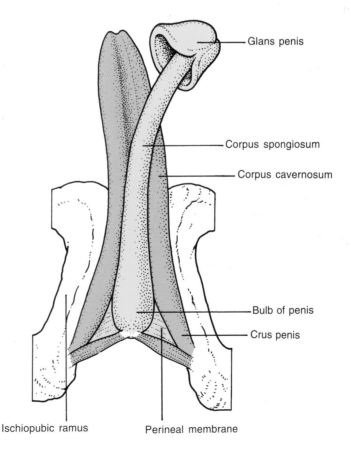

Fig. 27.6 **Roots of the penis in the superficial perineal pouch**

In the female, as in the male, the superficial perineal pouch contains the erectile tissues (Fig. 27.7). These are the two crura forming the *clitoris* and a paired structure on either side of the vestibule, the *bulb of the vestibule*. These erectile tissues are covered by thin muscles.

The perineum is supplied by the *internal pudendal artery* and the *pudendal nerve* (Fig. 27.7). These leave the pelvis through the greater sciatic foramen and enter the perineum through the lesser sciatic foramen (p.90). Their branching patterns are similar in the male and female. The anterior part of the skin is supplied by the *ilio-inguinal nerve* (L1).

Remove the skin and the superficial fascia and expose the structures in the superficial perineal pouch. In the male you may remove the scrotum and its contents if this is not done already.

Deep perineal pouch

This space is *deep* to the perineal membrane and contains a triangular sheet of skeletal muscle, the *deep transversus perineii* muscle. The middle part of the muscle surrounds the urethra forming the *external sphincter of the urethra*. The sphincter is formed by small-diameter fibres of the slow-twitch type which will exert a prolonged tone on the urethra to keep it closed. This part of the urethra is called the *membranous part of the urethra*. In the female, the deep transversus perineii muscle is pierced by the *urethra* and the *vagina*. The external sphincter is similar to that in the male.

Remove the contents of the superficial perineal pouch and the perineal membrane and expose the deep perineal pouch. Examine the deep transversus perineii muscle and the structures piercing it. Removal of the deep transversus perineii muscle should expose the undersurface of the pelvic diaphragm formed by the two levator ani muscles.

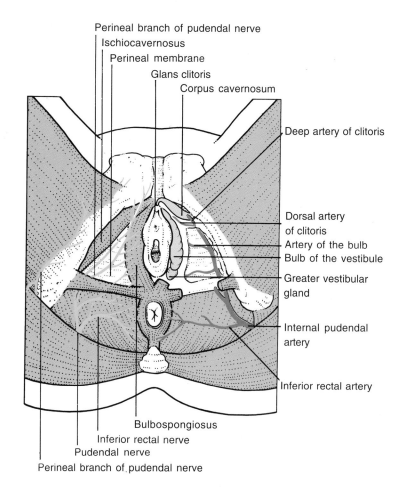

Fig. 27.7 **Dissection of the female perineum.** Arteries are shown on the left, and nerves on the right. The superficial muscles have been removed on the left to show the bulb of the vestibule and the greater vestibular gland

THE
BACK

28

The vertebral column, the spinal cord and the sacroiliac joint

Vertebral column

The vertebral column consists of:

- 7 *cervical* vertebrae
- 12 *thoracic* vertebrae
- 5 *lumbar* vertebrae
- the *sacrum* consisting of 5 fused vertebrae
- the *coccyx* formed by the fusion of four or more rudimentary vertebrae.

The vertebral column transmits the body weight on to the lower limbs through the sacroiliac joints. The spinal cord and its coverings and the spinal nerves are contained inside the vertebral canal.

Refer to Figure 28.1 and identify the parts of a vertebra.

Surface anatomy

The uppermost *spinous process* which is palpable is that of the 7th cervical vertebra. Palpate this and identify the spinous processes (spines) of the other vertebrae. The highest point of the iliac crest (p.58) is in line with the interval between L3–L4 spines. Identify this point.

> Remove the muscles from the posterior aspect of the vertebral column and expose the spinous processes and laminae of the vertebrae. Cut through the laminae of successive vertebrae on both sides using a bone forceps. Remove the laminae, the spinous processes and the remaining soft tissue en masse and expose the vertebral canal. Examine the epidural space.

The *epidural space* is the interval between the vertebrae and the dura mater of the spinal cord. It contains the small arteries which supply the spinal cord and the vertebral venous plexuses. The vertebral venous plexuses communicate with the veins draining the pelvic viscera, the breast and the thyroid gland. These veins are valveless and blood can flow in them in either direction depending on the pressure.

✳ Metastases from malignant tumours, in breast, thyroid gland and prostate, can reach the vertebrae through the vertebral venous plexuses which are connected to the veins draining these organs. Introduction of analgesic solutions into the epidural space (epidural anaesthesia) is commonly done in relieving pain during child birth.

✳ Exposure of the spinal dura, spinal cord and the nerve roots are done by a surgical procedure known as laminectomy. In this the spinal processes and the laminae are removed.

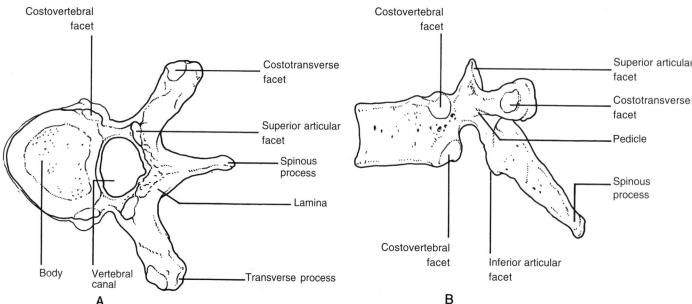

Fig. 28.1 **Typical thoracic vertebra: thoracic 7. A.** Superior view **B.** Lateral view

The arachnoid mater lines the inner surface of the dura mater. The subarachnoid space between the arachnoid and the pia mater contains cerebrospinal fluid (CSF). The pia mater closely covers the spinal cord.

Incise the dura and the underlying arachnoid mater and expose the spinal nerve roots (Fig. 28.2). Each *spinal nerve* is formed by a dorsal and a ventral nerve root. These lie in the *subarachnoid space* (Fig. 28.3). Define the two roots of the spinal nerves and also the *dorsal root ganglia*. Identify the *denticulate ligament*, a prolongation of the pia mater between the dorsal and ventral roots.

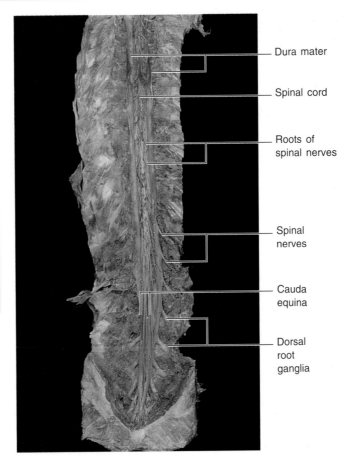

Fig. 28.2 **Vertebral canal, spinal cord and the spinal nerves**

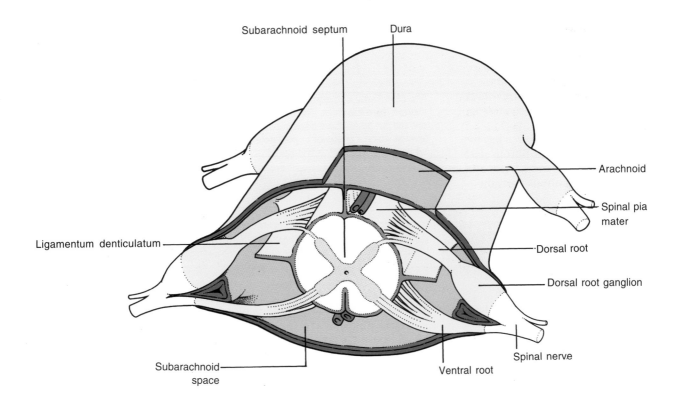

Fig. 28.3 **Spinal meninges**

Note that the spinal cord ends at the interval between the first and second lumbar vertebrae. The tapering end of the cord is the *conus medullaris*. From this a fibrous strand, the *filum terminale* extends to the coccyx. From the lower part of the cord, the lumbar and sacral nerves hang obliquely downwards. These nerves form the *cauda equina* (Fig. 28.4).

The *subarachnoid space* and the *cerebrospinal fluid* (CSF) extend into the upper half of the sacrum (in the sacral canal).

∗ A sample of CSF can be obtained by introducing a trochar and cannula into the subarachnoid space between the spinous processes of L3 and L4. This is at the level of the highest point of the iliac crest. As the spinal cord ends higher up, this procedure will not damage the cord.

Note that the spinal nerves leave the vertebral canal through the *intervertebral foramen*. On an articulated skeleton identify the boundaries of the intervertebral foramen. Anteriorly, the intervertebral foramen is bounded by the bodies of the adjoining vertebrae and the *intervening intervertebral disc*. Posteriorly it is bounded by the synovial joints between the two superior and the two inferior articular processes. Identify these boundaries on a radiograph (Fig. 28.5).

Each intervertebral disc has two parts. It has an outer fibrous part known as the *annulus fibrosus* and an inner more gelatinous part, the *nucleus pulposus*.

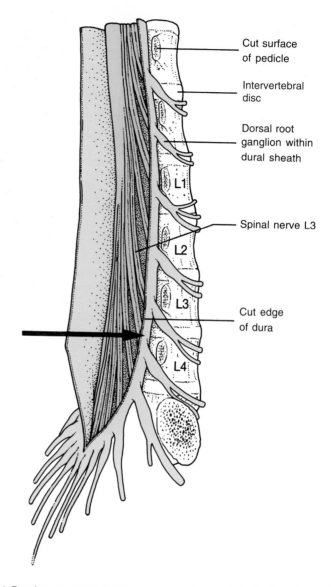

Cut surface of pedicle

Intervertebral disc

Dorsal root ganglion within dural sheath

Spinal nerve L3

Cut edge of dura

Fig. 28.4 **Dural sac surrounding the cauda equina, and the bodies of vertebrae T11–L5, viewed from the right.** The dura has been opened by a vertical cut down its posterior surface, and the cut edges have been separated to show the cauda equina. The arrow indicates the level at which a posterior or posterolateral protrusion of the L3–L4 disc can affect spinal nerve L4

∗ The nucleus pulposus may undergo degeneration, become brittle and can then herniate into the vertebral canal or into the intervertebral foramen. More commonly this happens in the lumbar part of the vertebral column and can cause back pain or back pain radiating to the leg (sciatica) by compression of the nerve roots.

∗ The spinal cord receives its blood supply from the anterior and posterior spinal arteries. These are branches of the intracranial part of the vertebral artery. The spinal arteries are reinforced by radicular arteries which enter the vertebral canal through the intervertebral foramen accompanying the spinal nerve roots. The radicular arteries which are branches of the cervical part of the vertebral, intercostal and lumber arteries are serially arranged. Damage to the radicular arteries from intercostal arteries in aortic surgery may result in ischaemia of the spinal cord (p.54).

Sacroiliac joint

The sacroiliac joint is a synovial joint. The body weight is transmitted from the sacrum to the ilium. The articular surfaces of the sacrum and the ilium are irregular and they fit together closely. The reciprocal irregularities of the articular surfaces and the strong ligaments make the joint stable for weight transmission.

Examine the articular surfaces of the sacrum and hip bone on isolated bones. Refer to Figure 28.6 and clean the *sacrotuberous*, *sacrospinous* and the *posterior sacroiliac ligaments*. Turn the specimen over and clean the anterior sacroiliac ligament. You may note that the posterior ligaments are stronger than the anterior one.

The weight of the body tends to rotate the upper part of the sacrum (*sacral promontory*) forwards, and the lower part and the coccyx backwards. These tendencies are prevented by the various ligaments of the joint.

Cut through the anterior sacroiliac ligament and try to separate the two bones. You will have to cut deeper into the joint as there is a very strong ligament, the *interosseus sacroiliac ligament*, inside the joint connecting the two bones. In an elderly person there may also be bony fusion between the bones making the separation more difficult.

✳ *Ankylosing spondylitis*, where there is new bone formation in the joint following inflammation, affects the sacroiliac joint and the joints between the vertebral bodies causing pain and stiffness.

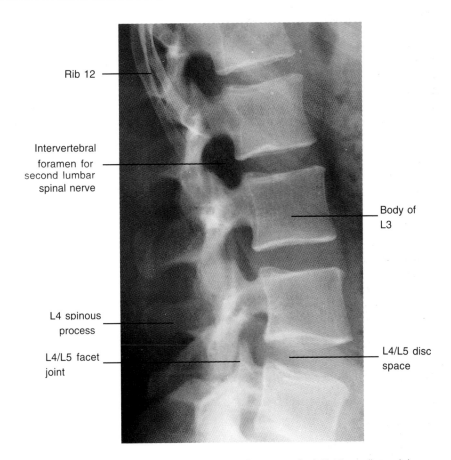

Rib 12

Intervertebral foramen for second lumbar spinal nerve

Body of L3

L4 spinous process

L4/L5 facet joint

L4/L5 disc space

Fig. 28.5 **Lateral radiograph of the lumbar spine in a normal adult.** The radiograph is centred on the body of L3

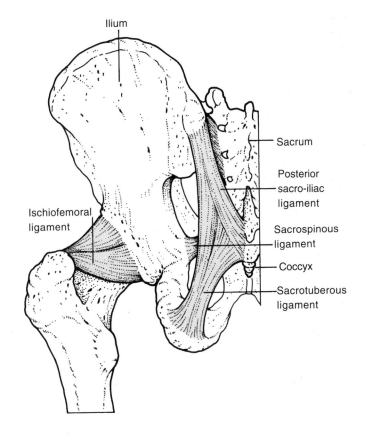

Ilium

Ischiofemoral ligament

Sacrum

Posterior sacro-iliac ligament

Sacrospinous ligament

Coccyx

Sacrotuberous ligament

Fig. 28.6 **Ligaments of the pelvis and femur: posterior view**

THE LOWER LIMB

29

The front and medial part of the thigh

OSTEOLOGY

Using Figures 29.1 A&B identify the following on a skeleton:

- the iliac crest
- the anterior superior iliac spine
- the anterior inferior iliac spine
- the posterior superior iliac spine
- the pubic tubercle
- the ramus of the pubis and ischium
- the ischial tuberosity
- the greater trochanter of femur
- the lesser trochanter of femur
- the linea aspera
- the adductor tubercle
- the medial and lateral condyles of femur
- the patella
- the medial and lateral condyles of tibia
- the tuberosity of tibia.

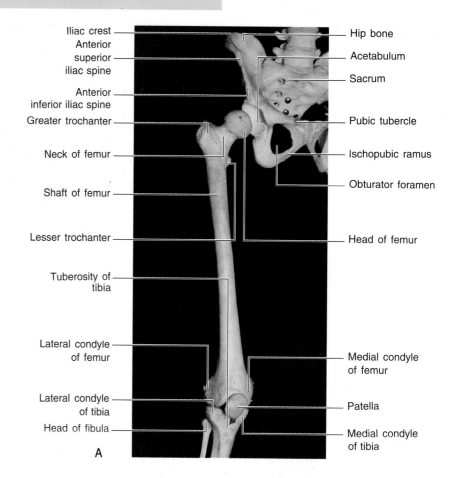

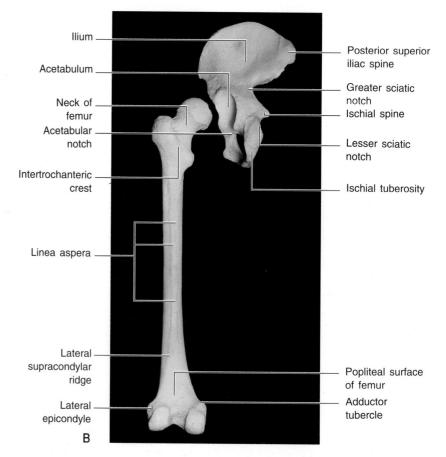

Fig. 29.1 **A. Bones of thigh and upper part of leg (anterior view) B. Hip bone and femur (posterior view)**

SURFACE ANATOMY

Palpate the structures labelled in Figure 29.2 on the cadaver and on yourself

Superficial structures

Make the following incisions:

1. from the anterior superior iliac spine to the pubic tubercle
2. from the pubic tubercle downwards skirting the external genitalia and along the medial aspect of the thigh as posteriorly as you can, to a point 15 cm below the knee joint
3. a transverse incision in the leg starting at the end of the last incision.

Carefully reflect the skin without removing the superficial nerves and vessels. In the superficial fascia expose and clean the great saphenous vein and its tributaries (Fig. 29.3). Note that at about 3.5 cms below and lateral to the pubic tubercle, the vein goes through an opening in the deep fascia, the *saphenous opening*, to join the femoral vein.

✳ The anatomy of the great saphenous vein and the venous drainage of the lower limb as a whole is of great clinical importance in relation to the production of varicose veins, venous thrombosis and venous ulcers. A blood clot (thrombus) from the vein can break loose and reach the lung through the right side of the heart. The dislodged thrombus is called an embolus. A large pulmonary embolus can cause sudden death.

✳ Most of the cutaneous nerves present in the superficial fascia are shown in Figure 29.3. Compression of the lateral cutaneous nerve of the thigh near the point where it enters the thigh causes pain and a tingling sensation along the lateral aspect of the thigh, a condition known as *meralgia parasthetica*.

The deep fascia of the thigh, the fascia lata, has a thick lateral aspect. This is the *iliotibial tract*, which extends from the iliac crest to the lateral condyle of the tibia. The iliotibial tract to which the gluteus maximus and the tensor fasciae latae are attached (see below) is an important structure in stabilising the knee joint. The iliotibial tract is taut when the slightly flexed knee is bearing the weight of the body as in the appropriate phases of walking and running.

Remove the superficial fascia retaining the great saphenous vein and examine the deep fascia and the iliotibial tract.

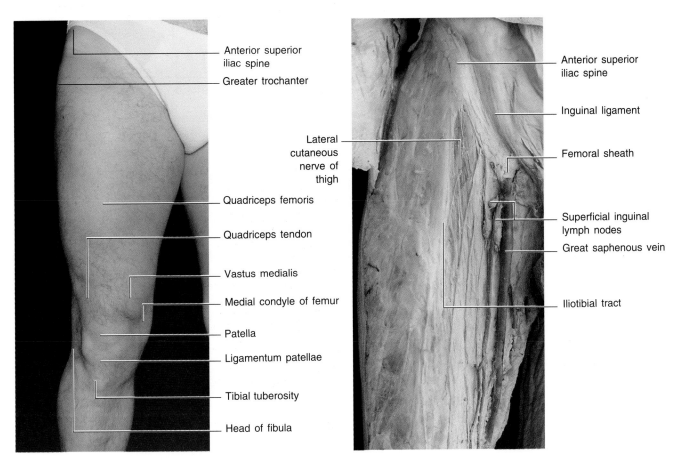

Anterior superior iliac spine

Greater trochanter

Lateral cutaneous nerve of thigh

Quadriceps femoris

Quadriceps tendon

Vastus medialis

Medial condyle of femur

Patella

Ligamentum patellae

Tibial tuberosity

Head of fibula

Anterior superior iliac spine

Inguinal ligament

Femoral sheath

Superficial inguinal lymph nodes

Great saphenous vein

Iliotibial tract

Fig. 29.2 **Front of thigh and upper part of leg**

Fig. 29.3 **Superficial dissection of thigh**

Femoral triangle

The femoral triangle is in the upper part of the front of the thigh. It is bounded laterally by the medial border of sartorius and medially by the medial border of the adductor longus, and above by the inguinal ligament (Fig. 29.4).

The femoral triangle contains from medial to lateral: the *femoral vein*, the *femoral artery* and the *femoral nerve* (Fig. 29.4). The femoral artery and vein are enclosed inside the *femoral sheath*. The femoral sheath has a potential space medial to the vein, the *femoral canal*. The femoral canal communicates with the abdominal cavity through the *femoral ring*.

✳ A *femoral hernia* can pass through the femoral ring into the femoral canal. The femoral ring is bounded laterally by the femoral vein, medially by the lacunar ligament which is a prolongation of the inguinal ligament on to the pubic bone, anteriorly by the inguinal ligament and posteriorly by the pectineus muscle.

Remove the deep fascia and expose the femoral triangle and the femoral sheath. Also clean the femoral nerve lateral to the femoral sheath. Open the sheath and expose the femoral vein and artery. Insert your little finger into the space medial to the vein and into the femoral ring and verify its borders.

✳ The *great saphenous* vein receives a number of tributaries corresponding to the superficial branches of the femoral artery (see below) just before it joins the femoral vein. This is an identification point to distinguish it from the femoral vein at operation. The femoral vein here has only one tributary: the great saphenous vein.

The great saphenous vein commences at the medial margin of the foot. The vein crosses in front of the medial malleolus. The constant position of the vein in front of the medial malleolus is used to expose the vein (cut down) to insert a cannula into it in an emergency.

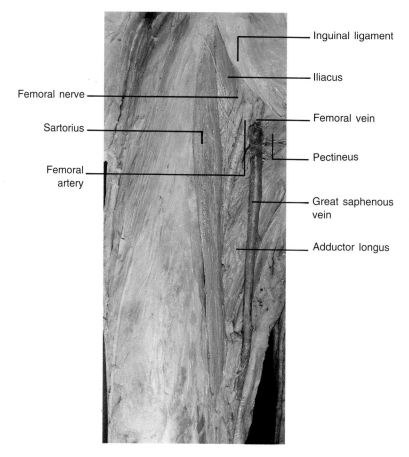

Femoral nerve

Sartorius

Femoral artery

Inguinal ligament

Iliacus

Femoral vein

Pectineus

Great saphenous vein

Adductor longus

Fig. 29.4 **Femoral triangle**

Clean the superficial branches of the *femoral artery*. The superficial epigastric goes upwards to the anterior abdominal wall, the superficial circumflex iliac goes towards the anterior superior iliac spine and the superficial external pudendal towards the pubic region. Identify and clean the *profunda femoris* branch of the femoral artery and also the *lateral* and *medial circumflex femoral arteries*.

Figure 29.5 summarizes the arterial supply of the lower limb. Occlusion of these arteries produces pain and gangrene in the limb.

✳ When the main artery is blocked an alternative pathway (*collateral circulation*) may open up through the various anastomoses shown in Figure 29.5.

Clean the branches of the *femoral nerve*. It is at a deeper plane and sometimes even posterior to the artery. It divides into its branches as soon as it enters the thigh.

✳ These anatomical variations make it a difficult nerve to block by injection of local anaesthetic agents.

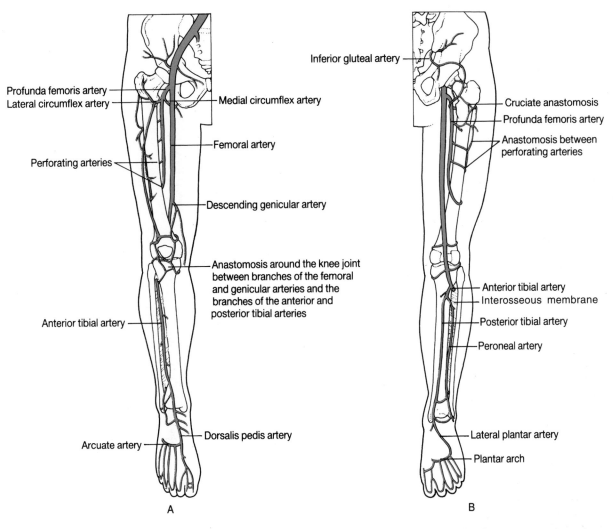

Fig. 29.5 **Summary diagrams showing the arteries of the lower limb. A.** Anterior view. **B.** Posterior view

The femoral nerve supplies the *pectineus*, the *sartorius* and the four parts of the *quadriceps femoris*, i.e. the *rectus femoris*, the *vastus lateralis*, the *vastus intermedius* and the *vastus medialis*. Trace these muscular branches as far as possible. Its sensory branches are the medial and the *intermediate cutaneous nerves of the thigh* and the *saphenous nerve*.

The saphenous nerve is the only branch of the femoral nerve extending below the knee joint. The nerve to rectus femoris is usually double, the upper nerve gives a branch to the hip joint. The nerve to vastus medialis is large. It continues down to supply the knee joint.

Examine the muscles forming the floor of the femoral triangle. From medial to lateral they are the *adductor longus*, *pectineus*, the *psoas major* and the *iliacus*. These muscles also form the anterior relations of the hip joint (p.120).

The adductor longus. This will be described with the muscles of the medial compartment of the thigh (p.167).

The pectineus. This takes origin from the ramus of the pubic bone. It is inserted into the upper part of the linea aspera. The femoral nerve supplies it. It helps in flexion and medial rotation of the thigh at the hip joint.

The psoas and iliacus. These are the major flexors of the hip joint. The psoas takes origin from the lumbar vertebrae, the details of which can be seen in the section on

the dissection of the abdomen (Fig. 22.6, p.79). The iliacus takes origin from the iliac fossa on the anterior surface of the ilium. Both the iliacus and the tendon of psoas pass deep to the inguinal ligament and enter the thigh. They lie in front of the capsule of the hip joint. The femoral artery lies in front of the tendon of the psoas. The two muscles are inserted together into the lesser trochanter of the femur. Beside flexion, the two muscles can also act as medial rotators of the hip. The iliacus is supplied by the *femoral nerve* and the psoas by *L1–L3 spinal nerves* in the abdomen.

Examine the sartorius muscle which extends from the anterior superior iliac spine to the medial condyle of the tibia. The sartorius is supplied by the femoral nerve. It is a flexor of the hip and knee and also, along with other long muscles connecting the hip bone to the leg, balances the hip bone on the femur.

Remove the middle third of the sartorius and moving the cut ends to the side, expose the underlying muscles (Fig. 29.6). Open up the space containing the femoral artery and the vein below the femoral triangle. This is the *subsartorial* or the *adductor canal*. It is also known as Hunter's canal (named after John Hunter).

Adductor canal

The adductor canal is the gutter-shaped groove bounded laterally by the vastus medialis and medially by the adductor longus above and the adductor magnus below. It contains the femoral artery, the femoral vein, the nerve to vastus medialis and the saphenous nerve.

Note that the femoral artery as it descends crosses from the lateral to the medial side of the femoral vein. The saphenous nerve crosses from the lateral side of the artery to its medial side. At all levels in the thigh, the artery lies between the saphenous nerve and the vein. This is in keeping with the medial rotation of the limb during development. The femoral artery and vein pass into the popliteal fossa from the adductor canal by passing through a hiatus in the adductor magnus. The saphenous nerve leaves the canal by passing along the posterior border of the sartorius and then accompanies the great saphenous vein as it descends in the leg.

Quadriceps femoris

The quadriceps femoris consists of the *rectus femoris*, the *vastus lateralis*, the *vastus intermedius* and the *vastus medialis*. It extends the knee joint. The rectus femoris, taking origin from the hip bone, is also a flexor of the hip joint. The other three components take origin from the femur and as such can act only on the knee. The *quadriceps tendon* is trilaminar; the tendon of the vastus lateralis is sandwiched between those of the intermedius and the rectus. The *patellar ligament* or the patellar tendon connects the lower border of the patella to the *tibial tuberosity*. The patella thus lies between two tendons

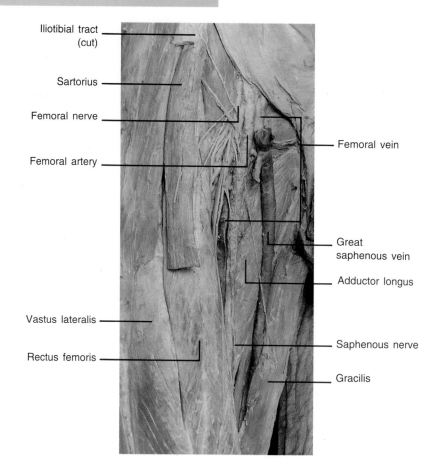

Fig. 29.6 **Contents of femoral triangle and the adductor canal**

Iliotibial tract (cut) — Sartorius — Femoral nerve — Femoral artery — Vastus lateralis — Rectus femoris — Femoral vein — Great saphenous vein — Adductor longus — Saphenous nerve — Gracilis

and is a *sesamoid bone*. Extensions of fibrous tissue from the quadriceps tendon to the condyles of the tibia are known as *patellar retinacula*. The quadriceps muscle, its tendon, the patellar ligament and the retinacula are all important factors stabilizing the knee joint.

Examine the vastus lateralis and the rectus femoris (Fig. 29.6). The former takes origin from the linea aspera of the femur. Cut the rectus femoris, reflect the cut ends and expose the vastus intermedius (Fig. 29.7). Clean the vastus medialis. Note that unlike the other members of the quadriceps, the vastus medialis is fleshy at its lower end and that these fibres lie horizontally as they attach to the patella. Study the quadriceps tendon through which the three vasti and the rectus femoris are inserted into the patella. Notice how they then insert into the tibial tuberosity through the patellar tendon.

✳ When the quadriceps contracts the patella moves *upwards* and *laterally*. Thus the patella has a tendency to dislocate laterally. The pull of the lower horizontal fibres of the vastus medialis is an important factor preventing such dislocation. Prominence of the lateral condyle of the femur and the patellar retinacula are additional factors stabilizing the patella.

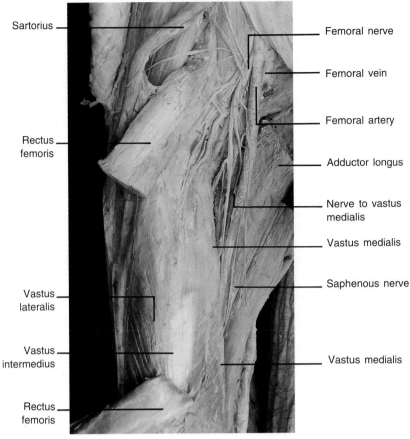

Sartorius

Rectus femoris

Vastus lateralis

Vastus intermedius

Rectus femoris

Femoral nerve

Femoral vein

Femoral artery

Adductor longus

Nerve to vastus medialis

Vastus medialis

Saphenous nerve

Vastus medialis

Fig. 29.7 **Adductor canal, quadriceps femoris, femoral nerve and femoral vessels**

Adductor muscles

Examine the *adductor longus*. Note that it has a tendinous origin from just below the pubic tubercle and that it is inserted into the *linea aspera* of the femur. Cut the adductor longus just below its origin, reflect it down and expose the *adductor brevis* (Fig. 29.8). Clean the anterior division of the *obturator nerve* on the surface of the brevis and trace its branches to the adductor longus, adductor brevis and the *gracilis*. The gracilis is a slender muscle connecting the pubic bone to the medial condyle of the tibia.

Now cut the adductor brevis in its upper third and reflect the cut ends to expose the *adductor magnus* and the posterior division of the obturator nerve. The latter supplies the adductor magnus and the *obturator externus* which is a muscle covering the external aspect of the obturator foramen. It can be exposed by removing the upper part of the adductor brevis and magnus from the pubis.

Adductor magnus

Origin: From the ramus of the pubis and ischium, and also from the ischial tuberosity.

Insertion: Into the linea aspera and the adductor tubercle of the femur.

As their names imply, the three adductor muscles move the thigh towards the midline at the hip joint (as you settle down on a car seat). They are also important in balancing while standing, preventing abduction. The adductor longus and brevis can also act as medial rotators of the thigh (preventing lateral rotation while standing). The part of the adductor magnus originating from the ischial tuberosity, along with the other hamstring muscles, extends the hip joint.

✱ The obturator nerve supplies all the muscles in the medial compartment of the thigh. It also supplies the hip and knee joint and hence pain produced in one joint can manifest as referred pain in the other. The nerve also supplies the skin of the medial part of the thigh. Therefore pelvic inflammation involving the obturator nerve can produce referred pain along the medial aspect of the thigh.

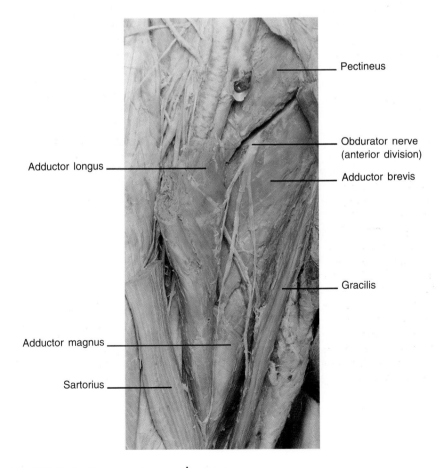

Adductor longus

Adductor magnus

Sartorius

Pectineus

Obdurator nerve (anterior division)

Adductor brevis

Gracilis

Fig. 29.8 **Adductor compartment of the thigh**

30

The gluteal region

Skin reflection

With the body in the prone position, make the following skin incisions:

1. along the iliac crest (if this is not done already)
2. a transverse incision along the upper part of the thigh
3. an incision joining (1) & (2) medially.

Reflect the skin and the superficial structures and expose the gluteus maximus muscle (Fig. 30.1).

Gluteus maximus

Origin. From the ilium behind the posterior gluteal line, the sacrum and the sacrotuberous ligament, a thick ligament extending from the ischial tuberosity to the sacrum.

Insertion. Major part into the iliotibial tract (p.103). The deeper portion into the gluteal crest of the femur.

Nerve supply. Inferior gluteal nerve.

Action. Powerful extension of the hip joint as in running and climbing stairs. It acts as an antigravity muscle controlling flexion as in sitting down from the standing posture. It is also a lateral rotator of the hip. Through the iliotibial tract it can extend as well as stabilize the knee joint.

Reflection of the gluteus maximus

Define well the upper and lower borders of the muscle. Insert your finger, or a blunt instrument, under these borders and separate the muscle from the underlying structures. Make a curved incision along the upper border of the muscle and reflect it downwards and laterally. Extreme care is needed in doing this to preserve the underlying structures, especially the inferior gluteal nerve and the posterior cutaneous nerve of the thigh. Refer to Figure 30.2 and identify the structures exposed.

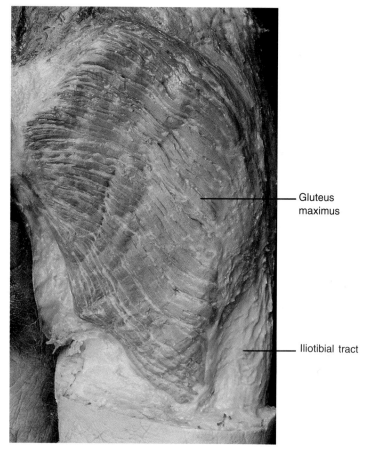

Gluteus maximus

Iliotibial tract

Fig. 30.1 **Gluteus maximus**

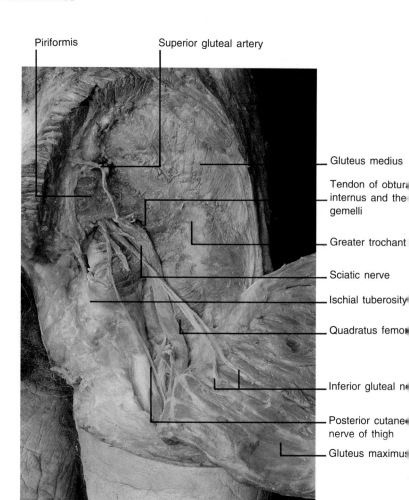

Piriformis

Superior gluteal artery

Gluteus medius

Tendon of obtura internus and the gemelli

Greater trochant

Sciatic nerve

Ischial tuberosity

Quadratus femo

Inferior gluteal n

Posterior cutane nerve of thigh

Gluteus maximus

Fig. 30.2 **Structures deep to the gluteus maximus**

Gluteus medius

Origin. From the gluteal surface of the ilium.

Insertion. Into the lateral surface of the greater trochanter.

Nerve supply. Superior gluteal nerve.

Action. Along with the gluteus minimus it can abduct the hip joint. When standing on one leg, gluteus medius and minimus of the supporting side prevent the hip from tilting to the unsupported side (it prevents adduction). When the muscles are paralysed, the tendency for tilting the pelvis to the unsupported side will be compensated by arching the trunk towards the supporting side.

Sciatic nerve (Fig. 30.3)

This is the largest nerve in the body and is formed in the sacral plexus (L4, 5, S1, 2, 3). It enters the gluteal region below the piriformis through the greater sciatic foramen. It supplies the muscles in the posterior compartment of the thigh and also all the muscles of the leg and foot. Its cutaneous branches supply the skin of the leg and foot except the skin along the medial border which is supplied by the saphenous nerve. The sciatic nerve in the lower third of the back of the thigh divides into the common peroneal and the tibial nerves. However, these two divisions of the nerve can remain separate almost throughout their course.

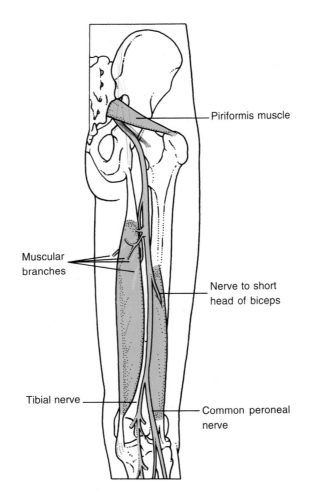

Fig. 30.3 **Course and distribution of the sciatic nerve**

(Labels: Piriformis muscle; Muscular branches; Nerve to short head of biceps; Tibial nerve; Common peroneal nerve)

Surface marking of the sciatic nerve. Palpate the posterior superior iliac spine, ischial tuberosity and the greater trochanter (p.102). Draw a line connecting the posterior superior iliac spine and the ischial tuberosity. The junction between the lower and middle third of this line is the point of entry of the nerve into the gluteal region. Join this to the midpoint between the greater trochanter and the ischial tuberosity and extend it vertically down to the lower third of the thigh. This marks the whole course of the nerve in the thigh.

Posterior cutaneous nerve of the thigh (S2, 3)

This supplies the back of the thigh and upper half of the back of the leg. It is derived from the same nerve root as the *pelvic splanchnic nerve* which supplies the pelvic viscera.

> ✳ Referred pain may sometimes be felt in pelvic inflammation along the back of the thigh and leg because of the common root value.

Short lateral rotators of the hip

These consist of the *piriformis*, the *obturator internus*, the *gemelli* and the *quadratus femoris*. All are inserted into the greater trochanter. Besides laterally rotating the thigh these muscles contribute to the fine adjustment and stabilization of the hip joint.

Inferior gluteal nerve and artery

The inferior gluteal nerve supplies the gluteus maximus. The branches of the artery anastomose with those of the femoral artery in the *cruciate anastomosis* just below the quadratus femoris muscle (Fig. 29.5, p.105).

Reflection of gluteus medius

Separate the muscle from the underlying gluteus minimus and detach the gluteus medius from its origin and reflect it laterally. The gluteus minimus will be exposed (Fig. 30.4). Clean the *superior gluteal nerve* and note that it supplies the *gluteus medius*, *gluteus minimus* and the *tensor fasciae latae* (see below).

Gluteus minimus

Like the medius, this takes origin from the gluteal surface of the ilium. It is inserted into the anterior aspect of the greater trochanter. It is supplied by the superior gluteal nerve and acts along with the gluteus medius (see above).

Tensor fascia lata

The gluteus medius anteriorly borders onto this muscle which takes origin from the anterior end of the iliac crest and is inserted into the iliotibial tract. Along with the gluteus maximus, this muscle exerts a pull on the iliotibial tract to extend and stabilize the knee joint. The tensor fasciae latae is supplied by the superior gluteal nerve.

✱ *Intramuscular injection.* Because of its muscle bulk, the gluteal region is a common site for intramuscular injections. To avoid damage to the sciatic nerve the injection should be given in the upper outer quadrant of the 'buttock'. The buttock is defined as the region extending from the iliac crest above, to the gluteal fold and greater trochanter below and is not just the most bulging part of the gluteal region.

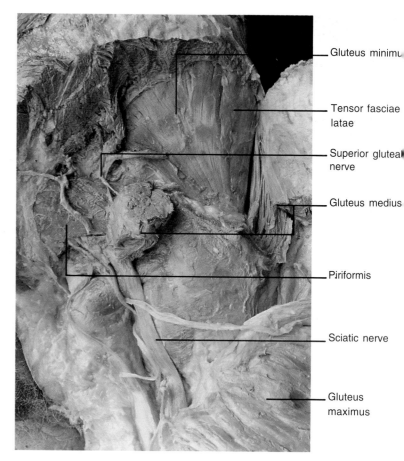

Gluteus minimus

Tensor fasciae latae

Superior gluteal nerve

Gluteus medius

Piriformis

Sciatic nerve

Gluteus maximus

Fig. 30.4 **Deep dissection of the gluteal region**

31

The back of the thigh and the popliteal fossa

Skin incision

Make a transverse incision in the middle of the calf and connect it to the cut end of the skin in the thigh by a vertical incision.

Reflect the skin and superficial structures and clean and identify the muscles of the back of the thigh (Fig. 31.1). These are the hamstring group of muscles.

Hamstrings

The hamstrings consist of the *biceps, semitendinosus, semimembranosus* and the hamstring part of *adductor magnus*.

Origin. Note that they have a common origin from the ischial tuberosity. The short head of the biceps takes origin from the linea aspera of the femur. Also verify the insertions of the hamstrings.

Insertion. The biceps into the head of the fibula, the semitendinosus and the semimembranosus into the medial condyle of the tibia and the adductor magnus into the adductor tubercle on the femur just above its medial condyle.

Nerve supply. The sciatic nerve.

Actions. They are flexors of the knee joint. When the knee is straight they limit flexion of the hip. They also have an extensor action on the hip joint especially when the position of the hip is intermediate between full flexion and full extension. This extension action is important in walking. The semitendinosus and semi-membranosus can medially rotate the flexed knee and the biceps can act as a lateral rotator.

Arterial anastomosis along the back of thigh (Fig. 29.5, p.105)

The four perforating arteries from the profunda femoris pierce the adductor magnus and reach the back of the thigh. These, along with branches from the inferior gluteal and the popliteal arteries, form a series of anastomoses along the back of the femur. These anastomoses act as collateral channels in cases of occlusion of the femoral artery.

Identify the sciatic nerve in the upper part of the thigh and trace its branches to the muscles. To get a better exposure of the nerve, detach the common tendon of origin of the semitendinosus and the biceps and reflect these laterally (Fig. 31.2). Note that the nerve divides into *common peroneal* and *tibial nerves* in the lower part of the thigh.

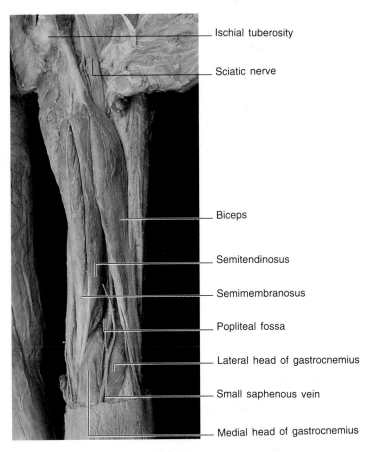

— Ischial tuberosity
— Sciatic nerve
— Biceps
— Semitendinosus
— Semimembranosus
— Popliteal fossa
— Lateral head of gastrocnemius
— Small saphenous vein
— Medial head of gastrocnemius

Fig. 31.1 **Muscles of the back of the thigh**

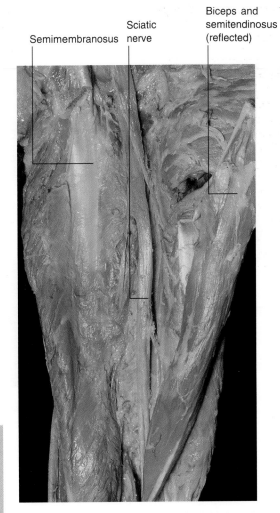

Semimembranosus   Sciatic nerve   Biceps and semitendinosus (reflected)

Fig. 31.2 **Sciatic nerve at the back of the thigh**

Popliteal fossa (Figs 31.3 & 31.4)

This is a diamond-shaped space behind the knee joint. It is bounded above by the tendon of the *biceps* laterally, the *semitendinosus* and *semimembranosus* medially and below by the *two heads of the gastrocnemius*. Its floor is formed from above downwards by the popliteal surface of the femur, the capsule of the knee joint and the *popliteus muscle*.

The popliteal fossa contains the *tibial* and the *common peroneal branches of the sciatic nerve*, the *popliteal artery* and the *popliteal vein*.

Surface anatomy

Bend your knee slightly and palpate the muscles forming the boundary of the popliteal fossa.

Remove the deep fascia and separate the muscles forming the upper boundary of the fossa and expose the contents. The *common peroneal nerve* lies along the posterior border of the tendon of the biceps. The *tibial nerve* lies in the midline. The *popliteal artery and vein* lie at a deeper plane. The vein here is often joined by the *short saphenous vein*. Clean the branches of the nerves and the artery.

Common peroneal nerve

Branches of the common peroneal nerve are:

- the peroneal communicating branch — of variable size, it joins the sural nerve in the leg to supply the lateral border of the foot
- the lateral cutaneous nerve of the calf which supplies the front and lateral aspect of the leg in its upper part
- the genicular branches which supply the knee joint.

✳ The common peroneal nerve winds round the neck of the fibula and divides into *superficial peroneal* and *deep peroneal nerves*. It is very superficial as it lies on the neck of the fibula and can easily be damaged in injuries of this region.

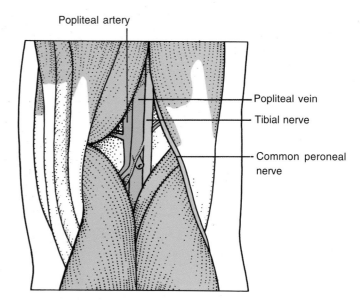

Fig. 31.3 **Popliteal artery, popliteal vein and the nerves in the popliteal fossa**

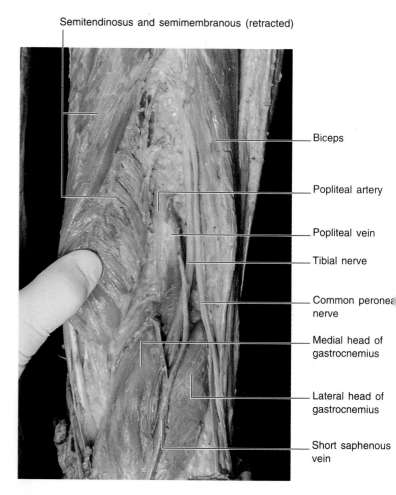

Fig. 31.4 **Popliteal fossa**

Tibial nerve

The tibial nerve lies in the midline and disappears after passing deep to the two heads of the gastrocnemius. It supplies all the muscles which take origin in the popliteal fossa, i.e. the two heads of the *gastrocnemius*, *plantaris*, *soleus* and *popliteus*. Its only cutaneous branch is the *sural nerve* which accompanies the short saphenous vein and supplies the lateral border of the foot. The tibial nerve also gives off three genicular branches.

Popliteal artery

The popliteal artery is the continuation of the femoral artery after it has passed through the hiatus in the adductor magnus. It lies deep in the popliteal fossa and is separated from the tibial nerve by the popliteal vein (Fig. 31.3). In its course in the popliteal fossa the artery lies, from above downwards: on the popliteal surface of the femur, the capsule of the knee joint and the popliteus muscle. The lower part, lying on the popliteus muscle, will be visible only at a later stage of the dissection (p.118). During its course in the popliteal fossa the artery gives off a number of muscular, genicular branches (to the knee joint) and its two terminal branches, the anterior and posterior tibial arteries (Fig.29.5, p.105).

The muscular branches supply to the two heads of the gastrocnemius. They are end-arteries and, if severed, will produce ischaemic necrosis of the heads supplied.

The genicular arteries are five in number (the upper and lower medial genicular, the upper and lower lateral genicular and the middle genicular arteries). The middle genicular artery pierces the posterior aspect of the capsule of the knee joint to supply the cruciate ligaments.

✳ The popliteal artery may be damaged in supracondylar fracture of the femur, especially if there is displacement of the lower fragment by the pull of the gastrocnemius.

✳ Being deeply placed, palpation of the popliteal artery pulsation is not easy. To feel the pulsation, the knee should be partially flexed, to relax the deep fascia and the finger tips inserted deeply into the centre of the popliteal fossa.

32

The front of the leg and dorsum of the foot

Skin reflection

Make the following incisions:

1. a vertical incision down the front of the leg and extend it to the dorsum of the foot up to the third toe
2. a transverse incision along the bases of the toes
3. a transverse incision across the ankle.
4. an incision on the dorsum of the big toe and on one of the other toes.

Remove the skin and the superficial fascia preserving the superficial peroneal nerve, the long saphenous vein and the saphenous nerve (Fig. 32.1). Note the thickening of the deep fascia in front of the ankle. This is the *extensor retinaculum* which holds the tendons of the muscles against the ankle joint and prevents them from bowstringing. Carefully remove the deep fascia and examine the muscles.

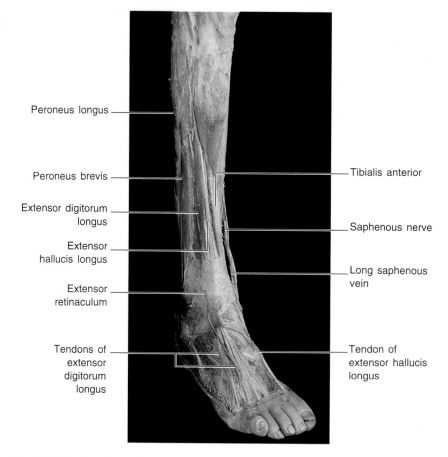

Peroneus longus

Peroneus brevis

Extensor digitorum longus

Extensor hallucis longus

Extensor retinaculum

Tendons of extensor digitorum longus

Tibialis anterior

Saphenous nerve

Long saphenous vein

Tendon of extensor hallucis longus

Fig. 32.1 **Structures in the front of the leg**

Long (great) saphenous vein

The vein is formed at the medial margin of the foot. It travels upwards in front of the *medial malleolus* and on the medial surface of the tibia, enters the thigh lying a hand's breadth behind the medial border of the *patella*, and terminates in the *femoral vein* in the upper part of the thigh after passing through the saphenous opening (p.103 & 104).

The deep veins, which accompany the arteries, are connected to the long saphenous vein by *perforating veins*. A number of such connections are present along the medial border of the leg. Through these, blood flows from superficial to deep veins as it is pumped upwards by the contraction of the calf muscles. Valves in the perforators prevent back flow of blood from the deep to the superficial veins.

> * When the valves are incompetent, the superficial veins will become varicose.

The long saphenous vein in the leg is accompanied by the saphenous nerve. This supplies the skin on the medial surface of the leg and foot up to the metatarsophalangeal joint of the big toe (the bunion region).

Tibialis anterior

Origin. From the interosseous membrane and the adjoining surface of the tibia.

Insertion. Into the medial cuneiform and the first metatarsal bone.

Tibialis anterior is a dorsiflexor of the foot at the ankle joint. Along with the *extensor hallucis longus* and the *extensor digitorum longus* it dorsiflexes the foot as the lower limb is carried forward during the *swing phase* of walking. This action prevents the toes catching the ground. It also applies the braking force to lower the limb onto the ground to initiate the *stance phase* of walking. Acting with the tibialis

posterior it inverts the foot (by which movement the sole of the foot is turned medially).

Extensor hallucis longus

Origin. From the fibula and the interosseous membrane.

Insertion. Into the base of the terminal phalanx of the big toe.

Extensor digitorum longus

Origin. From the fibula and the intermuscular septum lying between the muscle groups.

Insertion. Divides into four tendons which are inserted into the lateral four toes.

Peroneus tertius

Origin. From the lower part of the fibula.

Insertion. To the base of the fifth metatarsal bone.

All the muscles in the front of the leg are supplied by the *deep peroneal nerve* which accompanies the anterior tibial artery.

Separate the extensor digitorum longus and the extensor hallucis longus from the tibialis anterior and expose the deep peroneal nerve and the anterior tibial artery. The nerve lies lateral to the artery in front of the interosseous membrane (Fig. 32.2).

Anterior tibial artery

The anterior and posterior tibial arteries are terminal branches of the popliteal artery. The anterior tibial artery enters the front of the leg by passing over the upper border of the interosseous membrane. It descends lateral to the tibialis anterior. At the ankle, where its pulsation can be felt, it lies between the extensor hallucis longus and extensor digitorum longus. Beyond the ankle the artery is known as the *dorsalis pedis artery* whose pulsation may often be felt in the first interosseous space.

Deep peroneal nerve

The common peroneal nerve winds round the neck of the fibula and divides into the *superficial* and *deep peroneal* nerves. The deep peroneal nerve crosses deep to the extensor digitorum longus to reach the interosseous membrane whence it descends lateral to the anterior tibial artery. The nerve supplies the *tibialis anterior, extensor hallucis longus, extensor digitorum longus, peroneus tertius* and also *extensor digitorum brevis*, a small muscle on the dorsum of the foot. On the dorsum of the foot it pierces the deep fascia and supplies the *skin on the adjacent surfaces of the big toe and the second toe.*

Turn to the lateral aspect of the leg. Identify the *peroneus longus* and the *peroneus brevis* (Fig. 32.3). Trace the common peroneal nerve into the peroneus longus. Cut the muscle fibres covering the nerve and clean the nerve inside the muscle and note that it is dividing into its two terminal divisions, i.e. the superficial peroneal and deep peroneal nerves (Fig. 32.4).

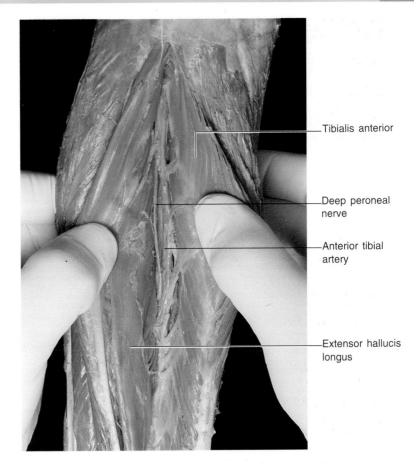

Fig. 32.2 **Deep dissection of the front of the leg (right side)**

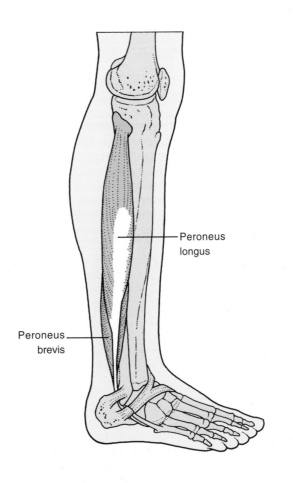

Fig. 32.3 **Peroneii: lateral view**

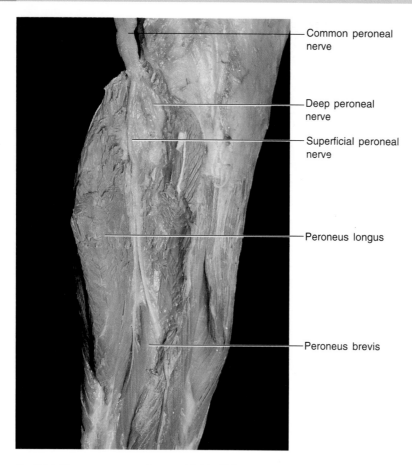

— Common peroneal nerve

— Deep peroneal nerve

— Superficial peroneal nerve

— Peroneus longus

— Peroneus brevis

Fig. 32.4 **Common peroneal nerve (right side)**

Peroneus longus

Origin. From the upper two-thirds of the lateral surface of the fibula.

The tendon lies behind the lateral malleolus, and crosses obliquely across the sole of the foot

Insertion. Into the medial cuneiform and the 1st metatarsal bone (see Fig. 36.5, p.129).

Peroneus brevis

Origin. From the lower two-thirds of the lateral surface of the fibula.

The tendon lies behind the lateral malleolus in front of the tendon of the longus.

Insertion. Into the styloid process at the base of the fifth metatarsal bone.

* In severe inversion injuries (foot being twisted inwards) tension on the peroneus brevis may produce avulsion of the styloid process of the fifth metatarsal bone into which the muscle is inserted.

Peroneus longus and brevis are supplied by the superficial peroneal nerve.

Peroneus longus and brevis evert the foot (lower the medial border so that the sole of the foot faces laterally) and also aid in plantar flexion. In standing, peroneus longus controls the sideways sway by pressing the medial side of the foot on to the ground. This action is better seen when standing on one leg when it prevents the body from falling to the unsupported side. The peroneus longus also plays an important role in maintaining the arches of the foot (p.127).

Superficial peroneal nerve

Besides supplying the two peroneii muscles, the superficial peroneal nerve supplies the skin on the lower part of the leg and the dorsum of the foot.

* The common peroneal nerve can be injured where it winds round the neck of the fibula. Complete paralysis of the nerve will result in loss of dorsiflexion and eversion of the foot and loss of sensation over the anterior aspect of the leg and dorsum of the foot. The plantar flexors of the foot will overact, producing a 'foot drop'. Patients tend to have a high-stepping gait because of the foot drop.

33

The back of the leg

Remove the remaining skin from the back of the leg. Dissect out the *short saphenous vein* and the *sural nerve* which accompanies it in its lower part. Identify these structures behind the lateral malleolus and clean them upwards. Expose the superficial layer of muscles as shown in Fig. 33.1.

Gastrocnemius

Origin. By two heads from the lateral and medial condyles of the femur.

Insertion. The tendon of the gastrocnemius fuses with the tendon of the soleus to form the *tendo calcaneus* or *tendo Achillis*. This tendon inserts into the posterior surface of the *calcaneus*.

Reflection of the gastrocnemius

Cut the two heads of the gastrocnemius from just below their origins and reflect the muscle downwards to expose the soleus and the plantaris (Fig. 33.2). The *plantaris* is a small muscle seen under the lateral head of the gastrocnemius and may be absent. Clean the branches of the tibial nerve which supply the two heads of the gastrocnemius and also the soleus and the plantaris.

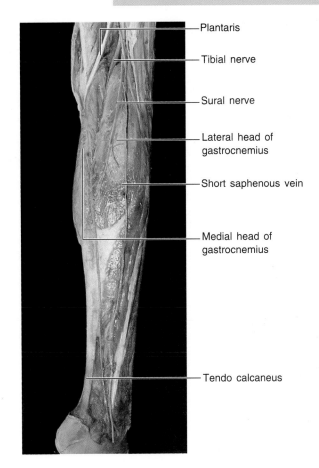

Fig. 33.1 **Superficial dissection of the back of the leg (right side)**

Plantaris

Tibial nerve

Sural nerve

Lateral head of gastrocnemius

Short saphenous vein

Medial head of gastrocnemius

Tendo calcaneus

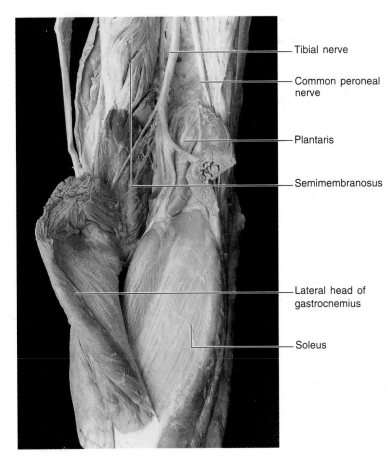

Fig. 33.2 **Structures under the gastrocnemius (right side)**

Tibial nerve

Common peroneal nerve

Plantaris

Semimembranosus

Lateral head of gastrocnemius

Soleus

Soleus

Origin. From the back of the fibula and tibia.

Insertion. See above.

Together with the gastrocnemius the soleus acts on the tendo calcaneus to produce *plantar flexion* at the ankle joint. These muscles give the driving force in walking, running and jumping. Soleus is an antigravity muscle and helps to maintain balance at the ankle in standing. *Perforating veins* from the superficial veins form a plexus in the soleus and these veins in turn are connected to the deep veins which accompany the deep arteries.

✳ Contraction of the muscle aids venous return. Stagnation in these veins predisposes to venous thrombosis and pulmonary embolism.

Plantaris

Origin. This muscle with a small belly takes origin from the lateral supracondylar area of the femur.

Insertion. Its long flat tendon is sandwiched between those of the gastrocnemius and soleus before it is inserted into the calcaneus.

Reflection of the tendo calcaneus

Cut the tendo calcaneus about 4 cm above its insertion Detach the soleus from its attachment to the fibula and reflect it laterally. This will expose the *flexor hallucis longus*, *flexor digitorum longus*, the *posterior tibial artery* and the *deep plantar nerve* (Fig. 33.3). Clean these structures. Clean the lower part of the popliteal artery and note its division into anterior and posterior tibial arteries.

Tendo calcaneus

The tendo calcaneus is the thickest and the strongest tendon in the body. It is able to withstand strains up to 10 tonnes. The arrangement of fibres in this gives it an elastic quality. When jumping, the body will land in an upright position with the foot held in plantar flexion by the contraction of gastrocnemius, soleus and plantaris. The strain is taken up by the tendo calcaneus which produces a recoil effect.

✳ The tendo calcaneus can be ruptured during games and severe exertions or sometimes following a trivial stumble. A precipitating factor may be poor blood supply to such a large tendon. If ruptured, on examination, a gap may be felt in the tendon, dorsiflexion of the ankle is exaggerated and plantar flexion is weak, the latter done only by the deep flexors.

Flexor hallucis longus

Origin. The flexor hallucis longus is a multipennate muscle taking origin from the flexor surface of the fibula and the interosseus membrane. It is the bulkiest and the most powerful of the deep muscles of the calf. The tendon of the muscle passes deep to the flexor retinaculum and lies on the under surface of the sustentaculum tali.

Insertion. Into the base of the distal phalanx of the big toe. It flexes the big toe and simultaneously plantar flexes the ankle thus giving forward momentum as the foot leaves the ground in walking. This muscle plays an important role in maintaining the medial longitudinal arch of the foot (p.127).

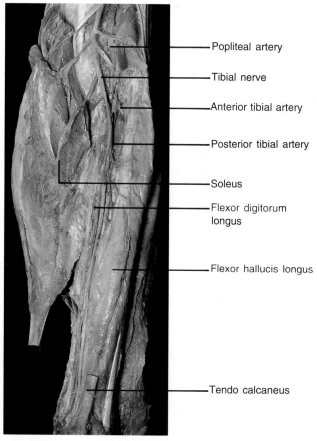

Popliteal artery

Tibial nerve

Anterior tibial artery

Posterior tibial artery

Soleus

Flexor digitorum longus

Flexor hallucis longus

Tendo calcaneus

Fig. 33.3 **Deep dissection of the back of the leg (right side)**

Flexor digitorum longus

Origin. The flexor digitorum longus takes origin from the posterior surface of the tibia. Its tendon passes through the flexor retinaculum to enter the sole of the foot. There it divides into four tendons each of which lie in the fibrous flexor sheath.

Insertion. The tendons of the digitorum longus pierce the tendons of flexor digitorum brevis and are inserted into the distal phalanx. The flexor accessorius muscle is inserted onto the tendon of the flexor digitorum longus. The *lumbrical muscles* take origin from the the four tendons of the muscle (p.128).

The flexor digitorum longus plantar flexes the lateral four toes and also the ankle joint. It pulls the toes downwards towards the ground to get the maximum thrust and grip during the toe-off phase in walking, running and jumping. Its tone maintains the longitudinal arch of the foot.

> Move the flexor hallucis longus laterally and expose the fascia covering the tibialis posterior muscle. Remove the fascia and expose the muscle.

Tibialis posterior

Origin. The tibialis posterior takes origin from the posterior surface of the tibia and fibula and from the *interosseus membrane.*

Insertion. Its tendon goes deep to the flexor retinaculum and is inserted mainly into the tuberosity of the navicular bone and by small slips into all the tarsal bones, except the talus, and also to the middle three metatarsal bones. The tibialis posterior plantar flexes the foot and also inverts it.

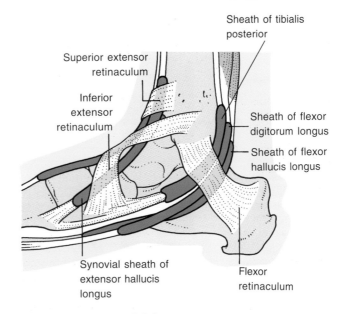

Fig. 33.4 Ankle region: medial view

Labels: Sheath of tibialis posterior; Superior extensor retinaculum; Inferior extensor retinaculum; Sheath of flexor digitorum longus; Sheath of flexor hallucis longus; Synovial sheath of extensor hallucis longus; Flexor retinaculum

Flexor retinaculum (Fig. 33.4)

The flexor retinaculum is a thickening of the deep fascia extending from the medial malleolus to the medial tubercle of the calcaneus. The structures deep to the retinaculum from anterior to posterior are as follows: tibialis posterior, flexor digitorum longus, posterior tibial artery, tibial nerve and the flexor hallucis longus.

> Incise the flexor retinaculum and examine the structures deep to it. Note that the artery and nerve divide into their lateral and medial plantar branches at this level. Clean the posterior tibial artery and the deep peroneal nerve and their branches

Tibial nerve

The tibial nerve in the posterior compartment of the leg is accompanied by the posterior tibial artery and they lie deep to the soleus between the hallucis longus and the digitorum longus.

Surface marking. The nerve is marked from the lower third of the thigh in the midline to behind the medial malleolus. It is the nerve of the posterior compartment and as such supplies all the muscles in this compartment. It gives off the medial calcaneal nerves to the skin of the heel.

Posterior tibial artery

The popliteal artery divides into the anterior and posterior tibial arteries at the lower border of the popliteus. The posterior tibial artery ends under the flexor retinaculum by dividing into lateral and medial plantar arteries. Its pulsation can be felt behind the medial malleolus. The artery in the leg gives off muscular branches and a nutrient artery to the tibia, as well as the peroneal artery. The *peroneal artery* starts about an inch below the commencement of the posterior tibial artery. It gives off a number of muscular branches, a nutrient artery to the fibula and a perforating artery which perforates the interosseus membrane and enters the extensor compartment.

34

The hip joint

Remove the adductor muscles and pectineus along with the femoral vein, artery and nerve from the front of the hip joint. The origin of the *obturator externus* muscle will be more fully exposed (Fig. 34.1). Remove the iliacus and the tendon of the psoas and look for a bursa underneath them which may often communicate with the joint. Examine the *iliofemoral* and *pubofemoral* ligaments (Fig. 34.2). Detach and remove also the obturator externus from its origin to expose the pubofemoral ligament more fully. This dissection will reveal the obturator nerve entering the thigh through the obturator foramen.

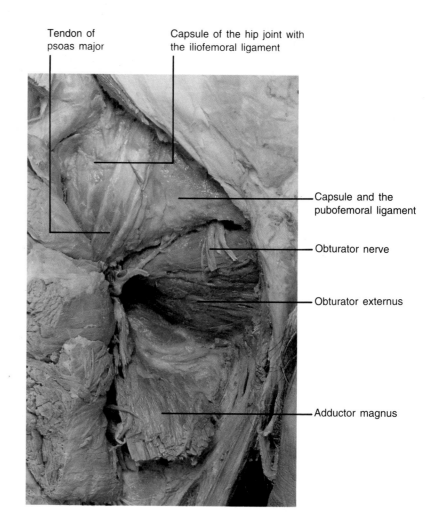

Tendon of psoas major

Capsule of the hip joint with the iliofemoral ligament

Capsule and the pubofemoral ligament

Obturator nerve

Obturator externus

Adductor magnus

Fig. 34.1 **Anterior aspect of the hip joint**

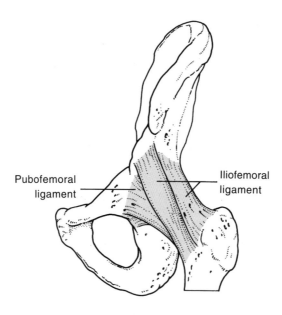

Pubofemoral ligament

Iliofemoral ligament

Fig. 34.2 **Hip joint: external view**

Turn the cadaver over and expose the posterior aspect of the joint. To do this remove the gluteus minimus, piriformis, the tendon of the obturator internus, the gemelli and the quadratus femoris along with the sciatic nerve. The posterior aspect of the capsule will now be visible. Note the insertion of the obturator externus into the *trochanteric fossa* of the femur (Fig. 34.3). Removal of the obturator externus might expose the *ischiofemoral ligament* more fully.

Turn the cadaver back to the supine position and cut and reflect the anterior part of the capsule exposing the interior of the joint. Identify the structures labelled in Figure 34.4. Using force if necessary, lever out the head of the femur from the acetabulum and examine its interior more fully (Fig. 34.5).

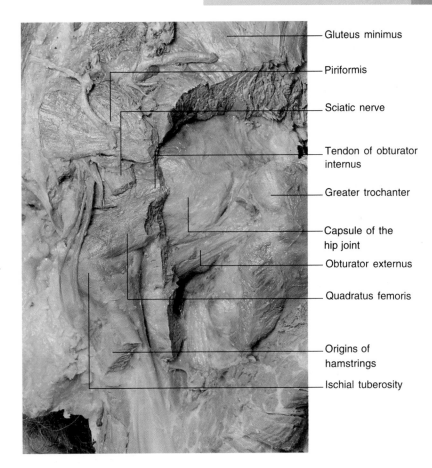

Fig. 34.3 **Posterior aspect of the hip joint**

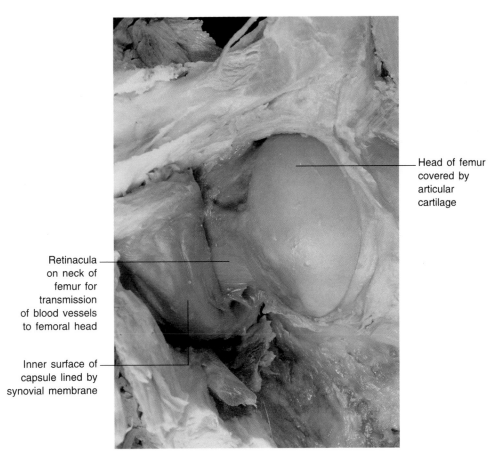

Fig. 34.4 **Interior of the hip joint**

As the lower limb should support the body weight in standing and also propel the trunk forward in locomotion the hip joint has to be more stable than the shoulder joint. The stability is achieved at the expense of mobility. The following factors stabilize the hip joint:

1. The *acetabular labrum*, a rim of fibrocartilage which deepens the acetabulum. As you might have noted the head fits tightly inside the acetabulum.
2. A strong capsule which is reinforced by the iliofemoral, pubofemoral and ischiofemoral ligaments.
3. Inside the joint there is the *ligament of the head of the femur* extending from the transverse ligament (bridging the acetabular notch) to the fovea on the head of the femur.

✳ The hip joint can be dislocated due to violent trauma as in a road traffic accident. *Posterior dislocation* is more common than anterior and central dislocations (where the head of the femur breaks through the acetabulum into the pelvis). The *sciatic nerve* is prone to injury in posterior dislocations.

✳ The head of the femur has a precarious blood supply. Most of the vessels enter the head through the retinacula which are reflections of the capsule and the synovial membrane onto the neck of the femur (Fig. 34.4). *Fracture of the neck of the femur,* which is a common injury in the elderly, can result in *avascular necrosis* of the head of the femur. In children, vessels accompanying the ligament of the head of femur are an important source of blood supply.

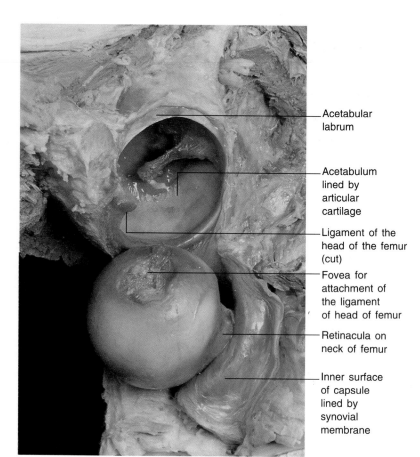

Acetabular labrum

Acetabulum lined by articular cartilage

Ligament of the head of the femur (cut)

Fovea for attachment of the ligament of head of femur

Retinacula on neck of femur

Inner surface of capsule lined by synovial membrane

Fig. 34.5 **Interior of the acetabulum**

35

The knee joint

The knee joint is the largest of the synovial joints. Within it the medial and lateral condyles of the tibia and the patella articulate with the femur. It has on its lateral aspect the *lateral (fibular) collateral ligament* covered by the tendon of biceps, on its medial aspect the *medial (tibial) collateral ligament* over which lie the gracilis, sartorius, and semimembranosus, posteriorly the *oblique popliteal ligament* and the popliteus muscle and anteriorly the *tendon of the quadriceps*, *patella* and the *ligamentum patellae*.

Examine again the quadriceps tendon, the patella and the ligamentum patella forming the anterior aspect of the joint (Fig. 35.1). These have been described already (p.106).

Turn to the lateral aspect of the joint. Cut the biceps just above the lateral epicondyle and turn it downwards to expose the cord-like *fibular collateral ligament*. Note that the ligament is attached to the lateral epicondyle above and to the head of the fibula below (Fig. 35.2).

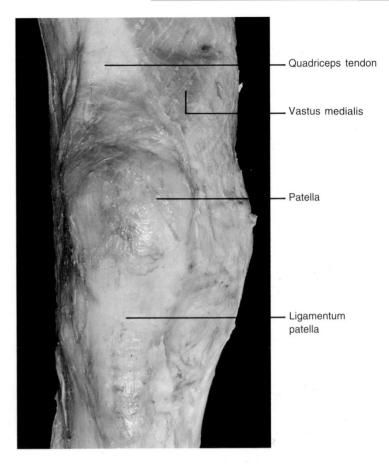

Fig. 35.1 **Anterior aspect of the knee joint (right side)**

- Quadriceps tendon
- Vastus medialis
- Patella
- Ligamentum patella

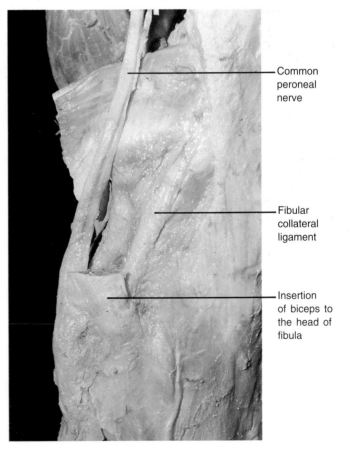

Fig. 35.2 **Lateral aspect of the knee joint (right side)**

- Common peroneal nerve
- Fibular collateral ligament
- Insertion of biceps to the head of fibula

Expose the *tibial collateral ligament* by detaching the insertions of sartorius, gracilis and semimembranosus. The ligament is broad and extends from the medial epicondyle of the femur to the medial surface of the tibia (Fig. 35.3).

Remove the nerves and vessels in the popliteal fossa. Cut and reflect the semimembranosus to its insertion and note the semimembranosus bursa deep to it. Remove the two heads of the gastrocnemius as well as the plantaris. Clean the posterior part of the capsule. The *oblique popliteal ligament* extending from the lateral side above to the medial side below will now be seen (Fig. 35.4). Also clean the popliteus which has a tendinous origin from the lateral condyle of the femur. Its fleshy fibres are inserted onto the tibia.

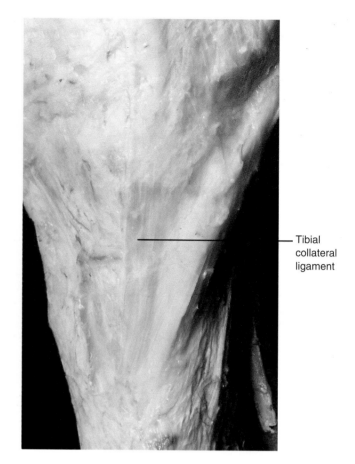

Tibial collateral ligament

Fig. 35.3 **Medial aspect of the knee joint**

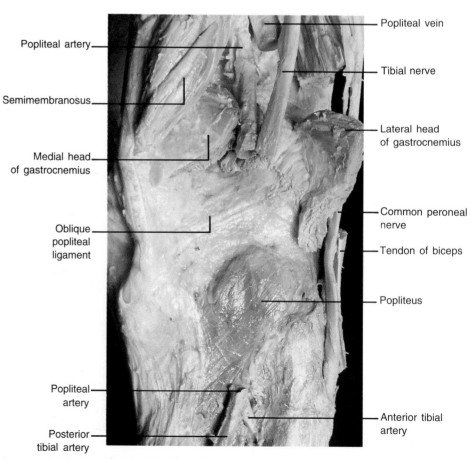

Popliteal artery

Semimembranosus

Medial head of gastrocnemius

Oblique popliteal ligament

Popliteal artery

Posterior tibial artery

Popliteal vein

Tibial nerve

Lateral head of gastrocnemius

Common peroneal nerve

Tendon of biceps

Popliteus

Anterior tibial artery

Fig. 35.4 **Posterior aspect of the knee joint**

Cut the quadriceps femoris transversely above the patella and reflect the lower end downwards. A synovial pouch, the *suprapatellar bursa*, will now be exposed. Note that it extends under the quadriceps and is continuous with the synovial cavity of the joint. Reflect the quadriceps tendon, patella and the patellar tendon further downwards and flex the knee joint. The *infrapatellar fold* of synovial membrane extending from the patellar ligament to the intercondylar area of the femur will now be exposed (Fig. 35.5). Cut the infrapatellar fold and flex the joint fully. The *anterior* and *posterior cruciate ligaments* and *medial* and *lateral menisci* will now come into view (Fig. 35.6). If necessary extend the incisions on each side of the patella to get a wider view.

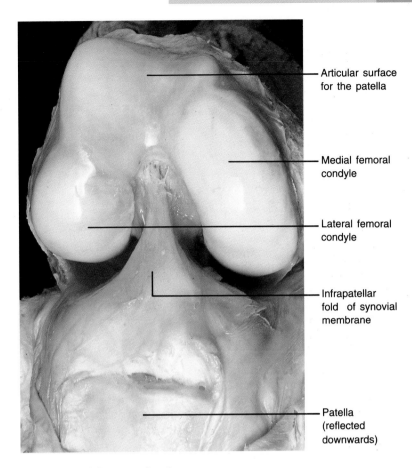

Articular surface for the patella

Medial femoral condyle

Lateral femoral condyle

Infrapatellar fold of synovial membrane

Patella (reflected downwards)

Fig. 35.5 **Interior of the knee joint—anterior view**

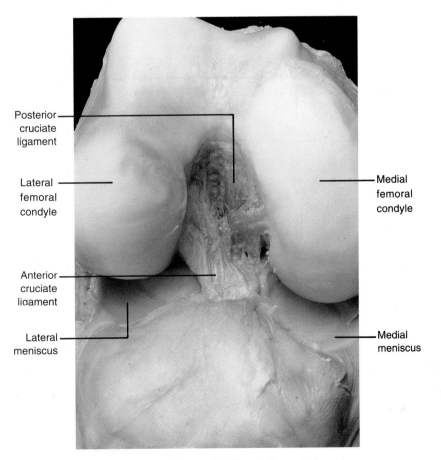

Posterior cruciate ligament

Lateral femoral condyle

Anterior cruciate ligament

Lateral meniscus

Medial femoral condyle

Medial meniscus

Fig. 35.6 **Interior of the knee joint: the cruciate ligaments—anterior view**

Cruciate ligaments

The *anterior cruciate ligament* extends from the anterior part of the intercondylar area of the tibia and is attached posteriorly to the lateral condyle of the femur.

> ✳ It prevents the femur from sliding excessively *backwards* on the tibia.

The *posterior cruciate ligament* extends from the posterior part of the intercondylar area of the tibia and it is attached anteriorly to the medial condyle of the femur.

> ✳ It prevents the femur from sliding excessively *forward* on the tibia.

Note that the cruciate ligaments are named after their tibial attachments.

> Extend the leg fully and note that the anterior cruciate ligament is taut. Flex the leg and verify that the posterior cruciate ligament prevents the anterior displacement of the femur on the tibia. Rotate the femur medially. The lateral collateral ligament will be taut and will limit the movement.
>
> Cut the lateral collateral ligament. Further medial rotation will now be possible. Cut the anterior cruciate ligament. Note that the femur can now be moved backwards on the tibia or the tibia forwards on the femur. Cut the posterior cruciate ligament. Detach the medial collateral ligament from the medial epicondyle and reflect it downwards and verify that this ligament is attached to the medial meniscus. The tibia can now be separated from the femur by cutting the remaining structures connecting the two bones. Examine the menisci and articular surfaces thus exposed.

Menisci

The menisci are tough avascular fibrocartilages whose anterior and posterior ends are anchored to the intercondylar area of the tibia. They deepen the concavity of the tibial surface and also helps to spread the synovial fluid.

> ✳ The *medial meniscus* is less mobile than the lateral meniscus and hence is more prone to injury. Its mobility is markedly restricted by its attachment to the tibial collateral ligament. The *lateral meniscus* is more circular and is attached to the popliteus which makes it more mobile and less prone to injury.

Movement of knee joint

Flexion and *extension* are the main movements of the knee joint. When the knee is fully extended the posterior part of the capsule and all the ligaments except the posterior cruciate ligament are taut converting the leg and thigh into a rigid column — the knee is '*locked*'. Flexion and extension of the tibia is accompanied by rotation; *medial rotation of the femur* during extension and lateral rotation during flexion. During flexion the *popliteus* will rotate the femur laterally loosening the ligaments to '*unlock*' the joint. Medial and lateral rotation can take place independently of flexion and extension in a fully flexed joint. Sartorius, semitendinosus, gracilis and semimembranosus rotate the tibia medially and the biceps rotates it laterally.

> ✳ The *patella* moves upwards during extension with a tendency for *lateral displacement* because of the pull of the quadriceps upwards and laterally parallel to the obliquity of the femur. Lateral dislocation of the patella is prevented by the prominence of the lateral condyle of the femur and by the horizontal fibres of the *vastus medialis* which are inserted onto the medial surface of the patella.

36

The sole of the foot

The foot is one of the most dynamic parts of the body. It provides physical contact with the ground and supports the body weight. Yet the foot is flexible and resilient enabling it to absorb shocks transmitted to it. The foot also provides the spring and lift during walking, running and jumping. All these functions are achieved by the segmented but arched configuration of the foot. For descriptive purposes the arches of the foot are divided into the *medial* and *lateral longitudinal arches* and the *transverse arch*. Each arch consists of a number of bones and joints and is supported by muscles and ligaments. The arches are maintained by the shapes of the bones, and the ligaments connecting them, as well as the muscles of the foot.

OSTEOLOGY

Refer to Figure 36.1 and identify the bones of the foot on an articulated skeleton.

The dissection of the sole of the foot is difficult and time consuming. In this session an attempt will be made to expose the major structures. It is not necessary to clean them meticulously.

The muscles of the sole of the foot are arranged in four layers and they are covered by the *plantar aponeurosis* which is a thickening of the deep fascia. The plantar aponeurosis and the muscles of the sole of the foot, extending from the proximal part of the foot to its distal part, act like tie beams or bowstrings, to maintain the longitudinal arches of the foot.

Remove the skin and superficial fascia from the sole of the foot and demonstrate the plantar aponeurosis (Fig. 36.2). This thickened middle portion of the deep fascia plays an important role in maintaining the longitudinal arches of the foot.

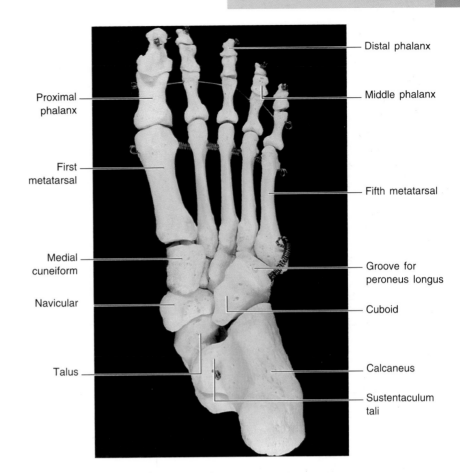

Fig. 36.1 **Bones of the foot: plantar aspect**

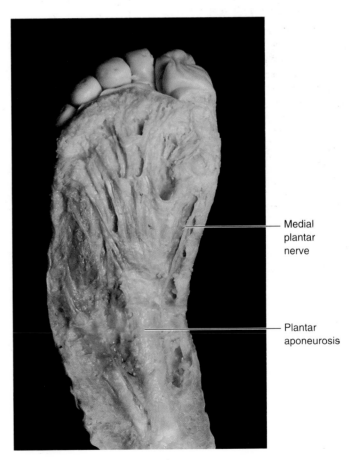

Fig. 36.2 **Superficial dissection of the sole of the foot**

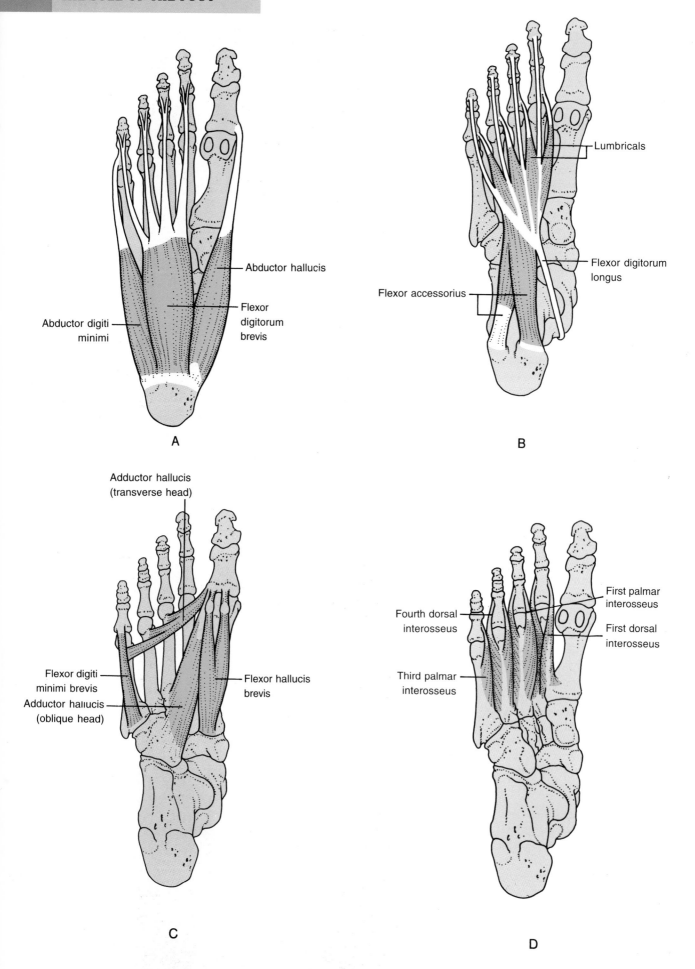

Fig. 36.3 **Sole of the foot. A.** First layer. **B.** Second layer. **C.** Third layer. **D.** Fourth layer

Removal of the plantar aponeurosis will expose the first layer of muscles. Figure 36.3 illustrates the layers of muscles and tendons in the sole of the foot.

Figure 36.4 illustrates the *lateral* and *medial plantar nerves* and *arteries* and their branches. The medial plantar nerve supplies the abductor hallucis, flexor hallucis brevis, flexor digitorum brevis and the first lumbrical. All the remaining intrinsic muscles including the adductor hallucis are supplied by the lateral plantar nerve. The cutaneous branches of the lateral plantar nerve supply the lateral third of the skin of the sole and the lateral 1½ digits. The sensory supply of the remaining skin is by the medial plantar nerve. Thus, the distribution of the two plantar nerves in the sole of the foot resembles the distribution of the median and the ulnar nerves in the palm of the hand.

Figure 36.5 illustrates the course and attachments of the *peroneus longus* on the sole of the foot. This lies in the fourth (deepest) layer along with the tibialis posterior. Note that the peroneus longus lies on the groove of the cuboid bone before reaching its insertion onto the medial cuneiform and the first metatarsal bone. The *tibialis posterior* is inserted into the tuberosity of the navicular bone and also into all the tarsal bones except the talus.

> Expose and study each layer of the sole of the foot by removing successive layers.

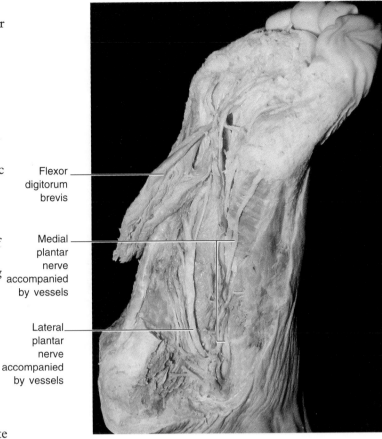

Flexor digitorum brevis

Medial plantar nerve accompanied by vessels

Lateral plantar nerve accompanied by vessels

Fig. 36.4 **Lateral and medial plantar nerves**

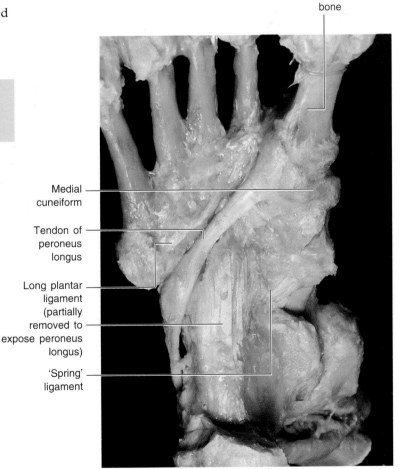

First metatarsal bone

Medial cuneiform

Tendon of peroneus longus

Long plantar ligament (partially removed to expose peroneus longus)

'Spring' ligament

Fig. 36.5 **Deep dissection of the sole of the foot**

37

The ankle joints and the joints of the leg and foot

Refer to Figure 37.1 and identify the bones of the foot on an articulated skeleton.

The tibia and fibula are connected to each other by the *superior* and *inferior tibiofibular joints* as well as by the *interosseus membrane*.

Open the superior tibiofibular joint and examine its articular surfaces. This is a synovial joint.

Identify the remaining muscles and tendons on the leg and foot and remove them. Examine the *interosseus membrane* connecting the tibia and fibula. Note how the anterior tibial artery enters the anterior compartment crossing the upper border of the interosseus membrane.

Clean the ligaments in the region of the ankle joint (Fig. 37.2). Identify the *deltoid ligament* and the *anterior* and *posterior talofibular* and the *calcaneofibular* ligaments of the ankle joint.

The synovial joint between the lower ends of the tibia and fibula and the talus is the *ankle joint*. *Plantar flexion* and *dorsiflexion* of the foot are the main movements in this joint. The *medial* and *lateral malleoli* which grip the sides of the *talus* along with the ligaments and the muscles crossing the joint stabilize the ankle joint.

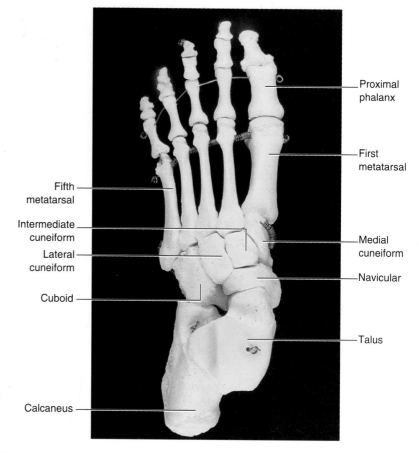

Fig. 37.1 **Bones of the foot: dorsal aspect**

Labels: Proximal phalanx, First metatarsal, Medial cuneiform, Navicular, Talus, Calcaneus, Cuboid, Lateral cuneiform, Intermediate cuneiform, Fifth metatarsal

Cut through the capsule and ligaments of the ankle joint and detach the talus (and the foot) from the leg bones. Examine the joint surfaces of the tibia and fibula and note how they, along with the malleoli, form a mortice to receive the talus. Open the *inferior tibiofibular joint* by cutting the interosseus tibiofibular ligament connecting the two bones. This is a *fibrous joint*.

Remove the muscles, tendons and nerves from the under surface of the foot and expose the *long plantar ligament* (Figs 37.2 & 37.3. This covers the under surface of the calcaneus and distally is attached to the cuboid and the central three metatarsal bones. It converts the groove on the cuboid into a tunnel in which the tendon of the peroneus longus lies. Clean the *plantar calcaneonavicular (spring) ligament*.

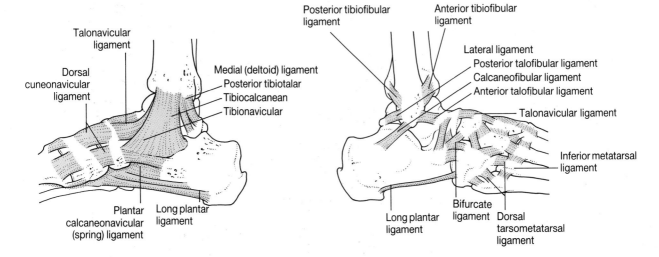

Fig. 37.2 **Ligaments of the foot and ankle. A.** Medial view. **B.** Lateral view

The spring ligament extends from the sustentaculum tali to the navicular bone. The head of the talus rests on its upper surface which forms part of the capsule of the subtalar joint.

Inversion and eversion take place in the *subtalar joint* where the talus articulates with the calcaneus and the navicular.

Remove the talus and open the subtalar joint by cutting the capsule and ligaments connecting the talus to the adjacent bones. The *interosseus talocalcaneal ligament* connects the talus to the calcaneus. Examine how the talus articulates with the calcaneus, the spring ligament and the navicular in the subtalar joint (Fig. 37.4).

The anterior surface of the head of the talus articulates with the navicular bone. This, along with the joint between the calcaneus and the cuboid (calcaneocuboid joint), form the *midtarsal joint*. Note that the medial component of the midtarsal joint (the talonavicular part) shares the same synovial cavity with the subtalar joint.

Inversion and eversion, which are twisting movements of the foot, enable one to walk on uneven ground. In eversion, the lateral border of the foot is slightly raised, making the sole of the foot face laterally. Inversion is the opposite movement, where sole of the foot faces medially. Most of these movements take place in the subtalar joint.

The tibialis anterior and the tibialis posterior invert the foot. Peroneus longus and brevis are the main evertors. As the muscles involved are attached beyond the midtarsal joint, in the early part of inversion and eversion the midtarsal joint also moves. In inversion the midtarsal joint adducts and in eversion it abducts. When the foot is on the ground, adduction of the forefoot is masked by lateral rotation of the leg. Similarly, eversion of a fixed foot is accompanied by medial rotation of the leg.

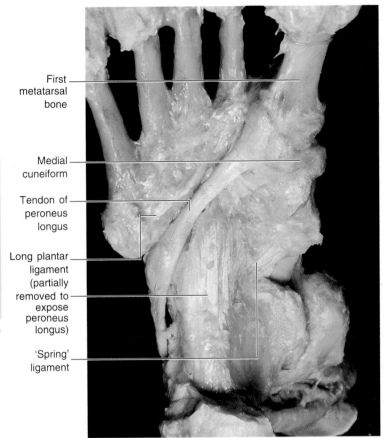

First metatarsal bone

Medial cuneiform

Tendon of peroneus longus

Long plantar ligament (partially removed to expose peroneus longus)

'Spring' ligament

Fig. 37.3 **Deep dissection of the sole of the foot**

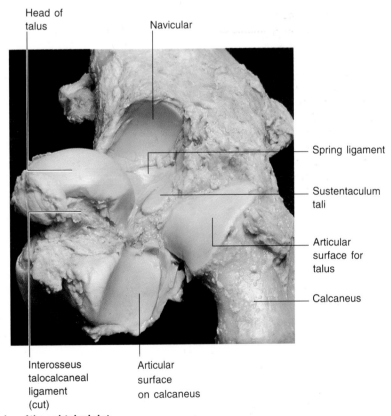

Head of talus

Navicular

Spring ligament

Sustentaculum tali

Articular surface for talus

Calcaneus

Interosseus talocalcaneal ligament (cut)

Articular surface on calcaneus

Fig. 37.4 **Interior of the subtalar joint**

THE HEAD AND NECK

38

The front of the neck

The front of the neck, or the anterior triangle, is defined as the region between the two sternocleidomastoid muscles. Here we will examine the thyroid gland, the carotid sheath and the infrahyoid muscles.

SURFACE ANATOMY

Refer to Figure 38.1 and identify the following on your partner:

- the two *sternocleidomastoid* muscles.

Feel in the midline, from above downwards:

- the *mandible*
- the *hyoid bone*
- the *thyroid cartilage*
- the *cricoid cartilage*
- the *tracheal rings*
- the *suprasternal notch*.

In the middle of the neck, in front of the sternocleidomastoid feel the pulsation of the common carotid artery. Note that the thyroid cartilage moves up and down with swallowing.

Skin reflection

Make a midline incision and reflect the whole of the skin from the front of the neck. In the superficial fascia define the *platysma* muscle. Reflect the platysma and as you do so look for the nerve supplying it. This is the cervical branch of the *facial nerve*. Review the attachments of the sternocleidomastoid (p.11). Identify the cut end of the spinal accessory nerve in the posterior triangle (p.11). Trace it proximally under the sternocleidomastoid and note that it supplies the muscle. Incise and remove the lower two-thirds of the sternocleidomastoid.

The lower border of the cricoid cartilage is an important level in the neck. It corresponds to the sixth cervical vertebra. It is the junction of the larynx and trachea and also that of the pharynx and oesophagus. At this level the carotid artery can be compressed against the transverse process of the C6 vertebra (carotid tubercle).

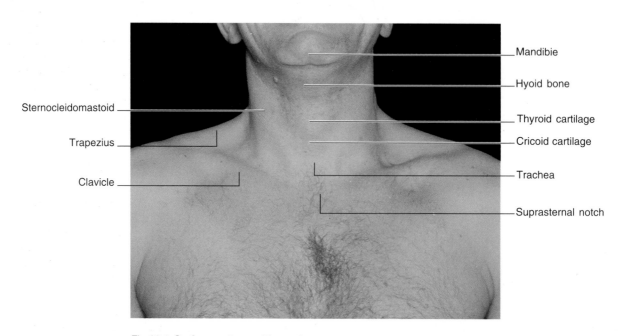

Sternocleidomastoid

Trapezius

Clavicle

Mandibie

Hyoid bone

Thyroid cartilage

Cricoid cartilage

Trachea

Suprasternal notch

Fig. 38.1 **Surface anatomy of the neck**

Refer to Figures 38.2 & 38.3 (also see Fig. 38.4) and clean the *infrahyoid muscles*, viz. the *sternohyoid, sternothyroid, thyrohyoid* and the *superior belly of the omohyoid*.

Define the *carotid sheath* covering the carotid arteries and dissect out the nerve loop, the *ansa cervicalis*, lying on the surface of the internal jugular vein. Trace its branches to the infrahyoid muscles. The carotid sheath contains the *internal jugular vein*, the *vagus nerve*, the *common carotid artery* and the *internal carotid artery*. Expose these structures. Trace the ansa cervicalis upwards and note that its superior limb originates from the *hypoglossal nerve*. Clean the hypoglossal nerve.

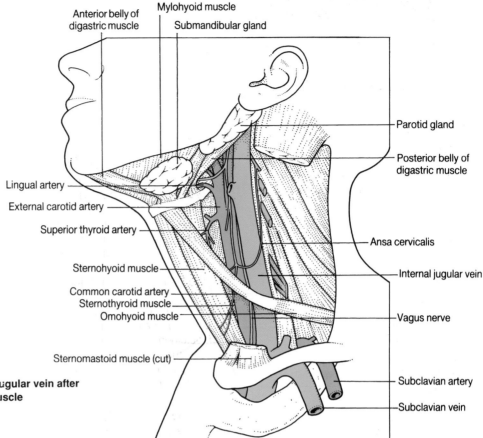

Fig. 38.2 Carotid arteries and internal jugular vein after removal of the sternocleidomastoid muscle

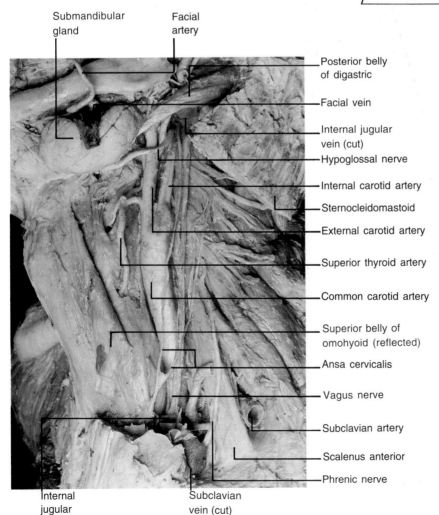

Fig. 38.3 Structures in the neck (internal jugular vein has been removed)

Infrahyoid muscles

The sternohyoid, sternothyroid and thyrohyoid connect the sternum, hyoid bone and thyroid cartilage. The omohyoid extends between the hyoid and the scapula. Contraction of the infrahyoid muscles prevent the *suprahyoid muscles* (connecting the hyoid to the mandible and the base of the skull) from elevating the hyoid. When the infrahyoids and the suprahyoids contract together the former group fixes the hyoid and the latter depresses the mandible (as in opening the mouth).

Common carotid artery

The right common carotid artery is a branch of the brachiocephalic trunk and the left is a direct branch from the arch of the aorta. At the upper border of the thyroid cartilage the common carotid artery divides into the *external* and the *internal carotid arteries*.

✳ The bifurcation can be at a higher level: a surgeon ligating the external carotid should be aware of this to avoid an inadvertent ligation of the common carotid.

The common carotid and the internal carotid arteries are enclosed by the carotid sheath in which the internal jugular vein lies lateral to the arteries, with the vagus nerve in-between the vein and the artery.

Internal jugular vein

The internal jugular vein is the major vein in the neck draining the pharyngeal veins, the facial vein and the thyroid veins. It starts at the base of the skull as a continuation of the sigmoid venous sinus and terminates behind the sternoclavicular joint by joining the *subclavian vein* to form the *brachiocephalic vein*.

✳ Internal jugular vein cannulation is carried out to measure the central venous pressure. The cannula is introduced into the internal jugular vein and advanced through the brachiocephalic vein and the superior vena cava into the right atrium. It is usually done on the right side as the above-mentioned veins lie in a straight line. The cannula is introduced by venepuncture at the middle of the anterior border of the sterno-cleidomastoid, immediately lateral to the carotid pulse. It can also be done at a lower level in the gap between the sternal and the clavicular heads of the sterno-cleidomastoid.

Thyroid gland (Figs 38.4, 38.5)

The thyroid gland has two *lateral lobes* connected by a midline *isthmus*. The gland is firmly bound to the larynx and trachea by the pretracheal fascia and hence moves with them during swallowing. The isthmus lies in front of the second, third and fourth tracheal rings. The *parathyroid glands* are embedded in the posterior surface of the lateral lobes. The thyroid gland is covered anteriorly by the infrahyoid muscles.

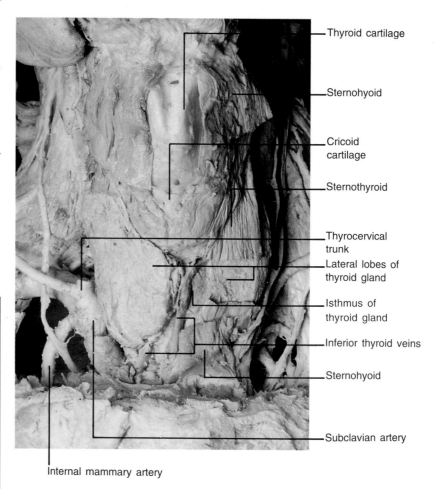

Thyroid cartilage

Sternohyoid

Cricoid cartilage

Sternothyroid

Thyrocervical trunk

Lateral lobes of thyroid gland

Isthmus of thyroid gland

Inferior thyroid veins

Sternohyoid

Subclavian artery

Internal mammary artery

Fig. 38.4 **Thyroid gland**

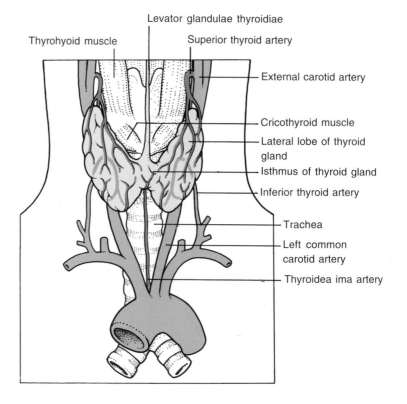

Thyrohyoid muscle

Levator glandulae thyroidiae

Superior thyroid artery

External carotid artery

Cricothyroid muscle

Lateral lobe of thyroid gland

Isthmus of thyroid gland

Inferior thyroid artery

Trachea

Left common carotid artery

Thyroidea ima artery

Fig. 38.5 **Thyroid gland: anterior view**

Cut the sternohyoid muscle just above the sternum and reflect it upwards. This will expose the underlying sternothyroid and the thyrohyoid more fully. Cut and reflect the sternothyroid and expose the thyroid gland.

Define the gland by removing its fascial coverings. Clean the isthmus and the lateral lobes and also look for the *pyramidal lobe* and the *levator glandulae thyroidiae* (which may be absent). Clean the *superior thyroid artery* and the accompanying superior thyroid vein. The former is a branch of the external carotid artery and the latter terminates in the internal jugular vein. Inferiorly, trace and clean the *inferior thyroid veins* which terminate in the left brachiocephalic vein. Look for a middle thyroid vein joining the internal jugular vein. The *inferior thyroid artery*, a branch of the thyrocervical trunk of the subclavian artery, lies deep to the carotid artery. Expose this by moving the common carotid artery and the accompanying internal jugular vein to the side or removing their lower part.

Identify the *oesophagus* behind the trachea. Look for the recurrent laryngeal nerve in the groove between the trachea and the oesophagus.

Recurrent laryngeal nerve

✳ The recurrent laryngeal nerve crosses the inferior thyroid artery very close to the thyroid gland (see p.149 Fig. 42.1). The nerve is vulnerable during ligation of the artery during thyroid surgery. The parathyroid glands are situated at the posterior aspect of the gland. In thyroidectomy (removal of the thyroid gland) the parathyroids are in danger of being removed, resulting in alteration of calcium and phosphorus metabolism.

✳ The recurrent laryngeal nerves supply the muscles of the larynx. A malignant tumour of the thyroid gland may compress the recurrent laryngeal nerve affecting the movements of the *vocal cords* resulting in a change in the voice. As mentioned already, the nerve is also prone to damage in thyroid surgery because of its close relation to the inferior thyroid artery.

Tracheostomy

✳ Tracheostomy is an operation done to keep the airway patent. In this, a hole is made in the trachea at the level of the second or third tracheal ring and a tracheostomy tube is introduced. The isthmus of the thyroid gland may have to be ligated and cut to expose the trachea. In a dire emergency an opening can be made through the cricothyroid ligament in the midline to maintain the airway. This is known as a 'cricothyroid jab' and may often be life-saving in an airway obstruction at or above the level of the vocal cords.

In the lower part of the neck, identify the *subclavian artery* and *subclavian vein*. Note that the *scalenus anterior* muscle lies in-between artery and vein (Fig. 38.3). Identify the *phrenic nerve* crossing the scalenus anterior muscle. Identify the *right vagus nerve*. Look for a branch of the right vagus, the *right recurrent laryngeal nerve*, given off as the vagus crosses the subclavian artery to enter the thorax. The right recurrent laryngeal nerve winds round the artery to reach the groove between the trachea and the oesophagus. On the left side look for the *thoracic duct* entering the left subclavian vein or the commencement of the left brachiocephalic vein. The thoracic duct has the calibre of a small vein, is thin walled and can be easily removed during dissection. It lies along the left border of the oesophagus before it terminates in the vein (Fig. 38.6).

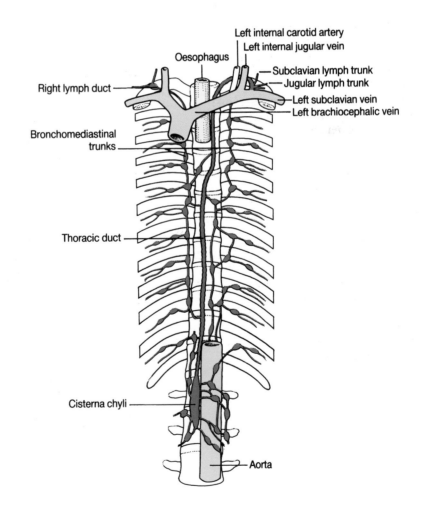

Fig. 38.6 **Cisterna chyli, thoracic duct and right lymph duct**

Finally, remove the subclavian vein to gain a better exposure of the subclavian artery. Clean the branches of the subclavian artery, viz. the *vertebral artery*, the *thyrocervical trunk* (giving off the inferior thyroid artery), the *internal mammary artery* and the *costocervical trunk* (Fig. 38.7).

The vertebral artery is the most important branch of the subclavian artery. It crosses the dome to the pleura, traverses the transverse foramina to the upper six cervical vertebrae and then turns posteriorly and medially over the posterior arch of the atlas to enter the cranial cavity through the foramen magnum by piercing the dura mater. The two vertebral arteries join to form the basilar artery. Branches of the vertebral artery and those of the basilar artery supply the brain and the spinal cord.

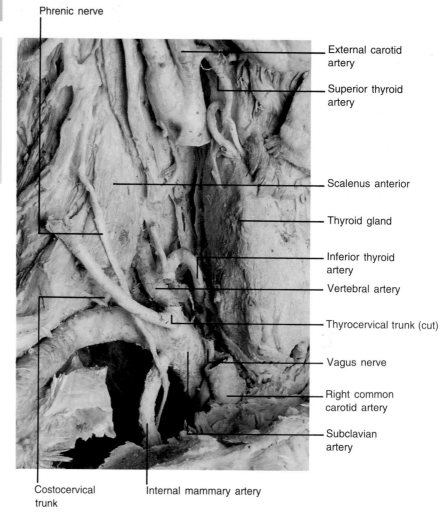

Phrenic nerve

External carotid artery

Superior thyroid artery

Scalenus anterior

Thyroid gland

Inferior thyroid artery

Vertebral artery

Thyrocervical trunk (cut)

Vagus nerve

Right common carotid artery

Subclavian artery

Costocervical trunk

Internal mammary artery

Fig. 38.7 **Blood supply of the thyroid gland and the branches of the subclavian artery**

39

The face, facial nerve, parotid gland and scalp

OSTEOLOGY

Refer to Figure 39.1 and identify the features of the anterior aspect of the skull and mandible.

Skin reflection

Reflect the skin of the face without damaging the underlying structures. The superficial muscles of the face and the muscles of facial expression are attached to the skin. Display of these muscles will be time consuming and should be attempted only if there is sufficient time. The muscles are illustrated in Figure 39.2.

Orbicularis oculi

Contraction of the orbicularis oculi muscle closes the eye. It has two parts. The *palpebral* part which arches across both the eyelids is used in blinking, and the *orbital* part which circumscribes the orbital margin is used in shutting the eye more forcefully as in 'screwing up the eyes'. Orbicularis oculi facilitates drainage of the lacrimal secretions (tears). The blinking action enables the lacrimal fluid to spread medially towards the nose. A few fibres of the orbicularis oculi are attached to the *lacrimal sac*, which dilates on contraction of the muscle thus sucking fluid into the sac. Elastic recoil of the sac empties the fluid into the nasal cavity through the *nasolacrimal duct*. The orbicularis oculi is supplied by the *facial nerve*.

✳ Paralysis of the orbicularis oculi as may occur in facial nerve paralysis will prevent the blinking action of the eyelid. This will fail to moisten the cornea and in turn lead to ulceration of the cornea.

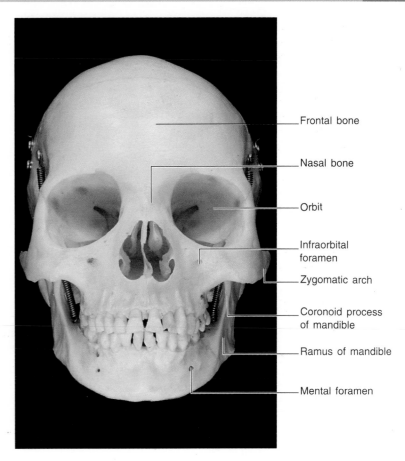

Fig. 39.1 **Skull and mandible: anterior view**

- Frontal bone
- Nasal bone
- Orbit
- Infraorbital foramen
- Zygomatic arch
- Coronoid process of mandible
- Ramus of mandible
- Mental foramen

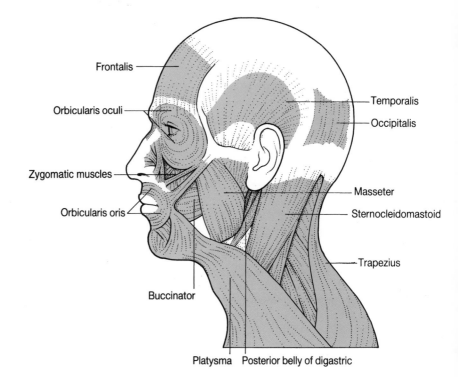

Fig. 39.2 **Muscles of the head and neck: lateral view**

- Frontalis
- Orbicularis oculi
- Zygomatic muscles
- Orbicularis oris
- Buccinator
- Platysma
- Posterior belly of digastric
- Temporalis
- Occipitalis
- Masseter
- Sternocleidomastoid
- Trapezius

Facial nerve

The facial nerve (seventh cranial nerve) leaves the skull through the stylomastoid foramen (Fig. 42.3, p.150) and enters the parotid gland where it divides into its terminal branches. These leave the gland along its anterior border to supply the muscles of facial expression and the buccinator muscle.

> Identify the parotid gland and dissect along its anterior border, thus exposing the branches of the facial nerve (Fig. 39.3).

The *temporal* branches of the facial nerve pass upwards to supply the frontalis muscle. The temporal and the *zygomatic* branches cross the *zygomatic arch* and supply the orbicularis oculi. The *buccal* branches, passing anteriorly, supply the buccinator (which is the muscle of the cheek and functions to push food medially from the space between the cheek and the teeth, i.e. the vestibule of the mouth). The *marginal mandibular* branch passes along the lower margin of the mandible to supply the muscles around the mouth, the *orbicularis oris*. The *cervical* branch passes downwards to supply the platysma.

> Trace the *facial artery* and the accompanying *facial vein* from the lower border of the mandible to the medial angle of the eye. Dissect out the *superficial temporal artery* and *vein* and the *auriculotemporal nerve* (a branch of the mandibular division of the trigeminal nerve) at the upper border of the parotid gland just in front of the auricle.

Parotid gland

The parotid gland is predominantly a serous salivary gland. It is situated below the external auditory meatus and extends onto the ramus of the mandible. It lies on the masseter and the sternocleidomastoid. The deep part of the gland is irregular in shape and extends almost up to the side wall of the pharynx and the carotid sheath, from which it is separated by the styloid process and its attached structures. The parotid gland is traversed by the facial nerve, the retromandibular vein and the external carotid artery in that order, from superficial to deep.

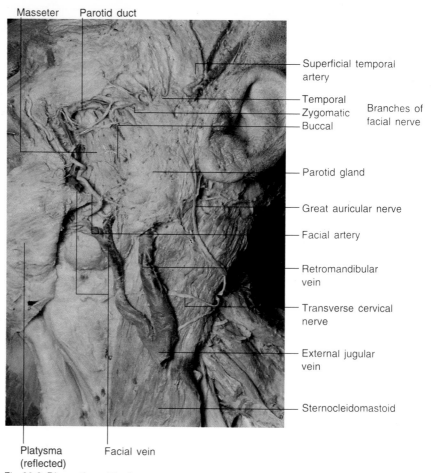

Masseter   Parotid duct

Superficial temporal artery

Temporal
Zygomatic — Branches of facial nerve
Buccal

Parotid gland

Great auricular nerve

Facial artery

Retromandibular vein

Transverse cervical nerve

External jugular vein

Sternocleidomastoid

Platysma (reflected)   Facial vein

Fig. 39.3 **Dissection of the face**

Clean the *parotid gland*. Identify the *parotid duct* in the middle of its anterior border. Trace the duct forward and note that it lies on the *masseter* muscle before piercing the *buccinator* to open in the vestibule opposite the upper second molar tooth. Trace the branches of the facial nerve back into the parotid gland by removing piecemeal the superficial part of the gland. Verify the terminal branches of the nerve in the substance of the gland. Trace the superficial temporal vein into the parotid gland and define the formation of the *retromandibular* vein by its union with the maxillary vein. Similarly, trace the superficial temporal artery into the gland and note that it is the terminal branch of the *external carotid artery*, the other branch being the *maxillary artery*.

✳ The parotid gland is enclosed inside a tough capsule derived from the investing layer of deep fascia of the neck. Mumps, a virus infection of the gland, is painful because the gland swells within the thick fibrous capsule.

A malignant tumour of the parotid gland unlike a benign mixed salivary tumour, may paralyse the facial nerve. The parotid duct and its branches can be demonstrated radiologically by injecting radio-opaque dye through the cannula inserted through the opening of the duct within the mouth.

Attempt to dissect out the sensory nerves of the face. They are derived from the *ophthalmic, maxillary* and *mandibular* divisions of the trigeminal nerve. The *auriculotemporal nerve* (mandibular division) has already been dissected. Lift the lower border of the orbicularis oculi and find the *infraorbital nerve* (maxillary division). Clear the fascia and muscle from the body of the mandible a third of the way from the midline and find the *mental nerve* (mandibular division). On the surface of the buccinator, embedded in the fat and fascia, is the *buccal nerve* (mandibular division). The dermatomes of the face are illustrated in Figure 39.4. Define these on your partner.

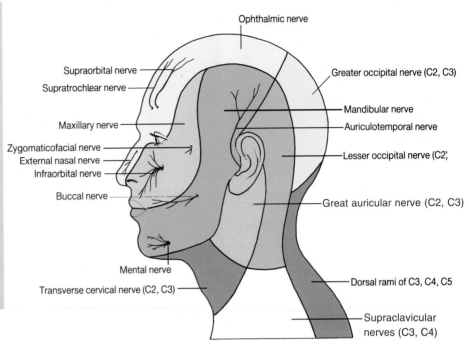

Fig. 39.4 **Sensory innervation of the head and neck**

Scalp

The scalp extends from the eyebrows to the *superior nuchal line* anteroposteriorly and to the zygomatic arches laterally. It consists of five layers:

- skin
- connective tissue
- aponeurosis of occipitofrontalis muscle
- loose areolar tissue
- periosteum.

Its composition can be remembered by using the five letters of the word S.C.A.L.P. as an acronym.

The skin of the scalp has an abundance of sebaceous glands and is the commonest site in the body for sebaceous cysts.

Remove the skin from the scalp and trace the *superficial temporal artery* and the *auriculotemporal nerve* from the face into the scalp. Similarly in front dissect out the *supraorbital* and *supratrochlear nerves* (Fig. 39.4) and the accompanying arteries (branches of the ophthalmic artery – internal carotid). At the back of the scalp attempt to dissect the *great occipital nerve* (posterior ramus of C₂) and the *occipital artery* (branch of the external carotid). Remove the connective tissue and define the frontal and occipital bellies of the *occipitofrontalis* (Fig. 38.2) and the aponeurosis connecting the two. This layer can now be peeled off along the loose areolar tissue to expose the *periosteum*.

✳ The scalp has an abundant blood supply, branches of the arteries coming from the external and internal carotid arteries. The vessels are embedded in the connective tissue and hence scalp injuries bleed profusely and often will require suturing. The layer of loose areolar tissue is continuous onto the eyelid below the orbicularis oculi and bleeding into this layer produces a 'black eye'.

✳ The veins of the scalp connect with the intracranial venous sinuses through emissary veins. An infection of the scalp may spread via this system producing meningitis and cranial venous sinus thrombosis.

40

The muscles of mastication, mandibular nerve and temporomandibular joint

Muscles of mastication

The muscles of mastication are the muscles attached to the skull and the mandible, viz. the *masseter*, the *temporalis*, the *lateral pterygoid* and the *medial pterygoid*. These muscles act on the *temporomandibular joint*.

Refer to Figures 40.1 and 40.2 and clean the *masseter*. This will require removal of all the structures lying over the masseter, including the parotid gland and its duct and the branches of the facial nerve. Note that the masseter extends from the *zygomatic arch* to the *ramus of the mandible*.

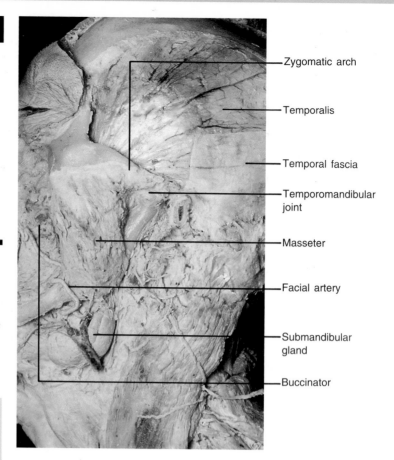

- Zygomatic arch
- Temporalis
- Temporal fascia
- Temporomandibular joint
- Masseter
- Facial artery
- Submandibular gland
- Buccinator

Fig. 40.1 **Muscles of mastication**

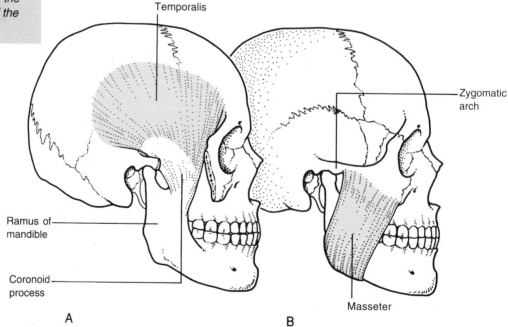

Temporalis

Zygomatic arch

Ramus of mandible

Coronoid process

Masseter

A

B

Fig. 40.2 **Temporalis and masseter muscles. A.** Temporalis. **B.** Masseter

Clean the surface of the *temporalis muscle*. Remove the temporal fascia covering the muscle. To expose the muscle more fully remove the anterior three-fourths of the zygomatic arch by cutting the bone with a bone-saw and bone forceps. Note the direction of the fibres of the temporalis. The posterior fibres are almost horizontal (Fig. 40.3). The temporalis has an extensive insertion to the coronoid process as well as to the *anterior border* of the ramus of the mandible.

The *lateral* and the *medial pterygoid muscles* lie deep to the ramus of the mandible (Fig. 40.4). These should be exposed by removing the ramus of the mandible without damaging the inferior alveolar nerve lying in the mandibular canal.

Cut the coronoid process of the mandible and reflect the temporalis muscle upwards to its origin from the temporal fossa. Remove the muscle completely to get a better exposure of the underlying structures. Similarly, remove the masseter from the ramus of the mandible and expose the surface of the bone fully.

Make a horizontal saw cut through the outer plate of the ramus at the angle of the mandible and another one at the lower part of the neck of the mandible. Make sure that these cuts are shallow. Do not saw through the whole thickness of the bone.

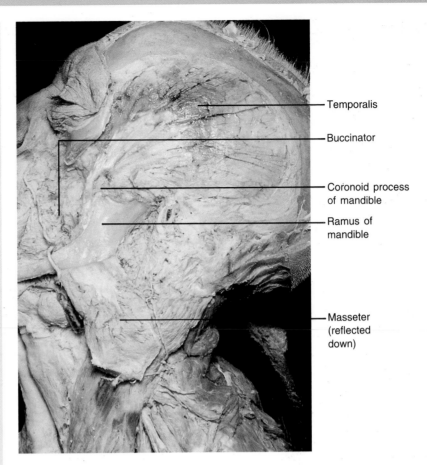

Fig. 40.3 **Temporalis muscle seen after removal of the zygomatic arch and after reflection of the masseter**

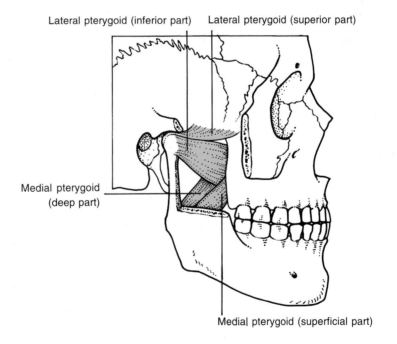

Fig. 40.4 **Pterygoid muscles**

Remove the outer plate of the ramus carefully using bone forceps. This will expose the *inferior alveolar nerve* within the bone. Remove the inner plate of the bone without damaging the nerve. The lateral and medial pterygoid muscles, which are medial to the ramus of the mandible, will now be exposed. Clean these muscles and expose the *lingual nerve* and the *maxillary artery* lying on their surface (Fig. 40.5). Look for the *chorda tympani* joining the lingual nerve from the posterior aspect. Clean the *inferior alveolar nerve* and identify a branch from it, the *nerve to mylohyoid*. Also trace the *buccal nerve* and see it emerging through the lateral pterygoid muscle.

Mandibular nerve

The mandibular division of the trigeminal nerve leaves the skull through the foramen ovale. The trunk of the nerve lies deep to the lateral pterygoid muscle and divides into an anterior and posterior division. Many of its branches have been exposed already. Besides the skin of the lower part of the face (p.141) the nerve gives sensory innervation to the lower teeth and gums, the cheek, the floor of the mouth and the tongue. The detailed distribution of the nerve is illustrated in Figure 40.6.

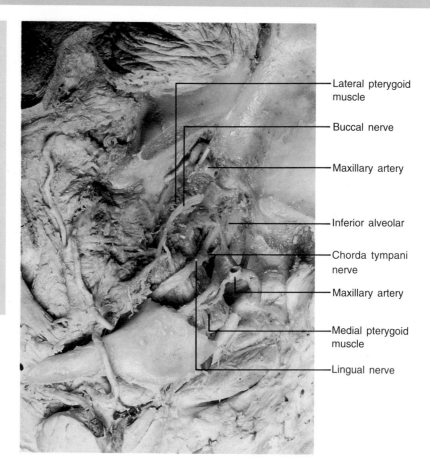

Lateral pterygoid muscle

Buccal nerve

Maxillary artery

Inferior alveolar

Chorda tympani nerve

Maxillary artery

Medial pterygoid muscle

Lingual nerve

Fig. 40.5 **Structures deep to the ramus of the mandible (left side)**

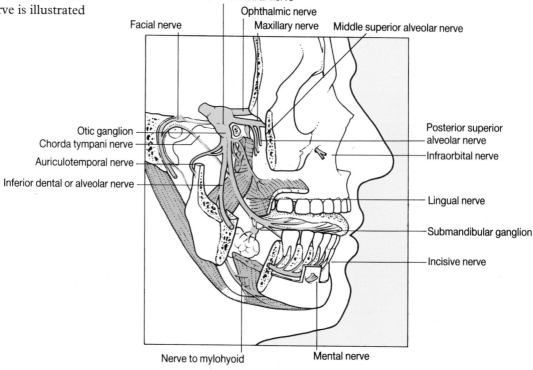

Facial nerve

Mandibular nerve
Ophthalmic nerve
Maxillary nerve   Middle superior alveolar nerve

Otic ganglion
Chorda tympani nerve
Auriculotemporal nerve
Inferior dental or alveolar nerve

Posterior superior alveolar nerve
Infraorbital nerve

Lingual nerve

Submandibular ganglion

Incisive nerve

Nerve to mylohyoid   Mental nerve

Fig. 40.6 **Deep dissection of the face, showing the distribution of the mandibular nerve (right side)**

Maxillary artery

The maxillary artery is a terminal branch of the external carotid artery given off in the depth of the substance of the parotid gland. It crosses the neck of the mandible to reach the lower border of the lateral pterygoid muscle. After crossing either superficial or deep to the muscle the artery enters the *pterygopalatine fossa*. Most of its branches are distributed along with those of the mandibular and maxillary nerves (Fig. 40.7).

Middle meningeal artery

The middle meningeal artery, a branch of the maxillary artery, enters the skull through the *foramen spinosum* to supply the dura mater and the periosteum.

❋ Rupture of this vessel is common in head injuries and will result in an *extradural haemorrhage*.

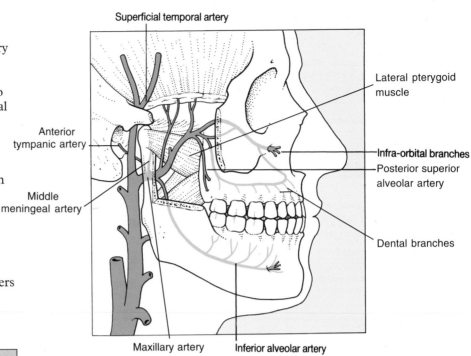

Fig. 40.7 **Maxillary artery and its branches**

Temporomandibular joint (Fig. 40.8)

At this synovial joint, the head of the mandible articulates with the mandibular fossa at the base of the skull. The two surfaces are separated by an *intra-articular disc*. The head of the mandible does not lie in the coronal plane, but has its medial end a little posterior to the lateral one. The disc is firmly bound to the medial and lateral extremities of the head.

Define the insertion of the lateral pterygoid muscle to the capsule of the temporomandibular joint. The tendon pierces the capsule and is inserted into the upper part of the neck of the mandible and to the articular disc. Cut through the capsule of the joint and remove the head of the mandible and the articular disc from the mandibular fossa. Study the shape of the condyle of the mandible and the overlying disc.

Reflect the lateral pterygoid muscle with the head of the mandible forward. Clean the trunk of the mandibular nerve and its two divisions deep to the lateral pterygoid muscle.

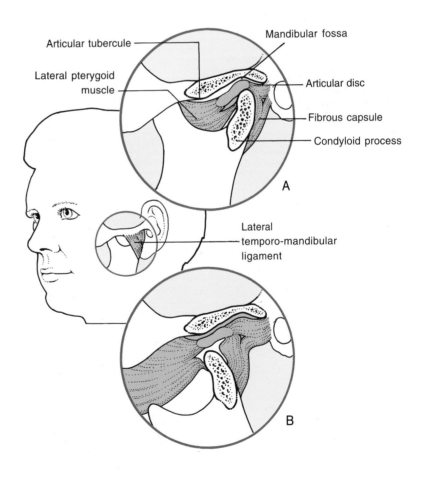

Fig. 40.8 **Left temporomandibular joint, sagittal sections. A.** Mouth closed. **B.** Mouth open

41

The submandibular region

Submandibular salivary gland

The submandibular salivary gland is situated in a triangular area bounded by the *anterior* and *posterior bellies of the digastric muscle* and the mandible (Figs 41.1 & 41.2).

Clean the structures on the surface of the submandibular gland. Note that the *facial vein* and often the *marginal mandibular branch of the facial nerve* cross the surface of the gland. Trace the *facial artery* from the external carotid through the posterior part of the gland till it reaches the mandible.

Clean the anterior and posterior bellies of the digastric muscle. Note its intermediate tendon attached to the hyoid bone. Remove, if necessary, the superficial part of the submandibular gland to expose the underlying structures.

✳ When the submandibular gland is affected by calculus (stone) or tumour this gland is excised. The operation is carried out through a skin incision below the jaw. the marginal mandibular branch of the facial nerve can be damaged by this incision. The incision is usually placed more than 2.5 cm below the angle of the jaw to preserve the nerve.

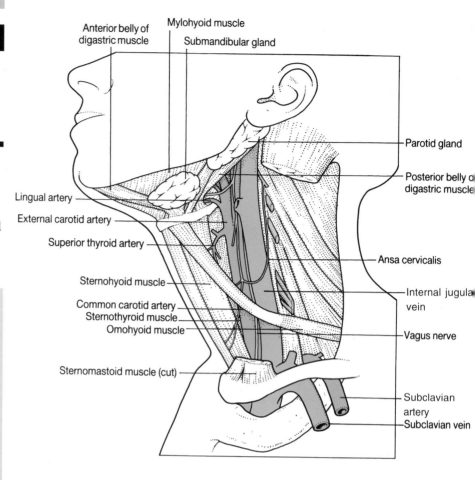

Fig. 41.1 **Submandibular gland and the structures in the neck**

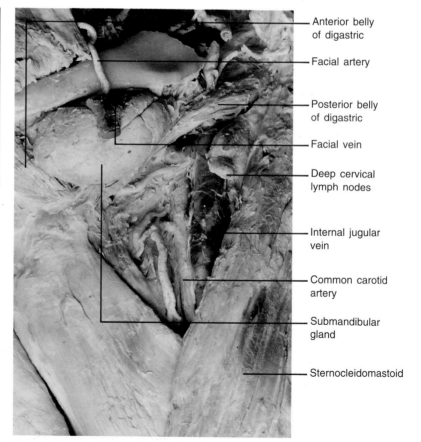

Fig. 41.2 **Submandibular region**

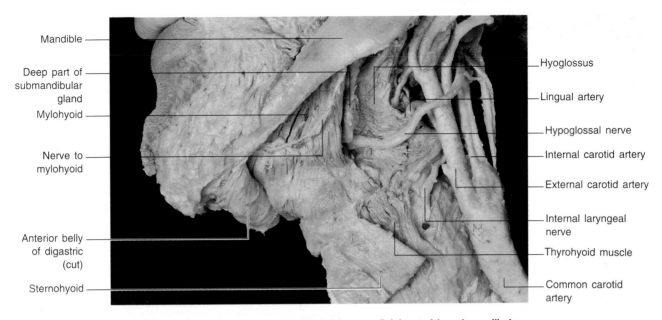

Mandible

Deep part of submandibular gland

Mylohyoid

Nerve to mylohyoid

Anterior belly of digastric (cut)

Sternohyoid

Hyoglossus

Lingual artery

Hypoglossal nerve

Internal carotid artery

External carotid artery

Internal laryngeal nerve

Thyrohyoid muscle

Common carotid artery

Fig. 41.3 **Submandibular region after removal of the superficial part of the submandibular gland and the digastric muscle**

Define the *stylohyoid muscle* accompanying the posterior belly of the digastric. Identify the *mylohyoid muscle.* To get a better view of the muscle cut the intermediate tendon and reflect the digastric muscle. Clean the *nerve to the mylohyoid* (a branch of the inferior alveolar nerve) on the surface of the mylohyoid muscle (Fig. 41.3). This nerve supplies the mylohyoid and the anterior belly of the digastric muscle. The posterior belly of the digastric and the stylohyoid are supplied by the facial nerve.

The mylohyoid muscle at each side unite in the midline to form the floor of the mouth. Above the mylohyoid lies the mouth or oral cavity; below it lies the neck.

Suprahyoid muscles (Fig. 41.4)

The suprahyoid muscles, consisting of the mylohyoid, the digastric, the stylohyoid and the geniohyoid (which lies deep to the mylohyoid) function as a group. They are important in depressing the mandible against resistance as in chewing food which has a sticky consistency. For this the hyoid bone should be fixed and this is done by the infrahyoids (p.135). The suprahyoids can also elevate the hyoid bone and the larynx. This happens during swallowing. The two mylohyoids, with the raphe between them, form the floor of the mouth. Their contraction helps to elevate the tongue in swallowing.

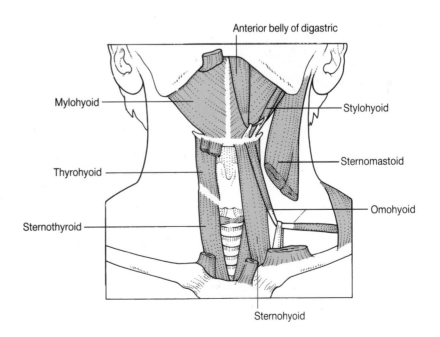

Anterior belly of digastric

Mylohyoid

Thyrohyoid

Sternothyroid

Stylohyoid

Sternomastoid

Omohyoid

Sternohyoid

Fig. 41.4 **Suprahyoid and infrahyoid muscles.** Note that the superficial muscles have been removed on the right side of the neck

Hypoglossal nerve

Trace the hypoglossal nerve lying on the surface of the carotid arteries and note that it lies on the hyoglossus muscle (a muscle of the tongue) before disappearing under the mylohyoid. On the hyoglossus the nerve divides into branches which supply the muscles of the tongue.

✳ The hypoglossal nerve is seldom damaged. Section of the nerve paralyses the affected half of the tongue, which appears shrunken and wrinkled. If the tongue is protruded it deviates towards the paralysed side. (The unopposed action of the genioglossus of the opposite side makes the tip of the tongue deviate towards the paralysed side.) In patients with facial nerve palsy, the hypoglossal nerve may be cut and sutured to the distal end of the facial nerve to restore facial muscle tone and some movement.

Hyoglossus muscle

The hyoglossus muscle which forms the side of the tongue (p.168) lies in a plane deep to the mylohyoid. The borders of the two muscles overlap. The deep part of the submandibular gland lies between the mylohyoid and the hyoglossus. The part of the gland being deep (superior) to the mylohyoid (floor of the mouth) is in the oral cavity. The submandibular duct emerges from the deep part of the gland to open on either side of the midline under the tongue.

Reflection of the mylohyoid

Cut the attachment of the mylohyoid to the hyoid bone and reflect the muscle forward to expose the structures in the floor of the mouth. Clean the hypoglossal nerve and the *deep part of the submandibular gland* which are now exposed more fully (Fig. 41.5). Look for the *submandibular duct* and the sublingual gland anterior to the deep part of the submandibular gland. Trace the *lingual nerve* (p.144) to the hyoglossus. Look for the *submandibular ganglion* on the lingual nerve.

Lingual nerve

The lingual nerve supplies the anterior two-thirds of the tongue. The parasympathetic fibres (secretomotor) supplying the submandibular and sublingual glands and the minor salivary glands on the tongue synapse in the submandibular ganglion attached to the lingual nerve. The preganglionic fibres from the facial nerve reach the lingual nerve via the *chorda tympani nerve* (see Fig. 40.6, p.144).

Clean the *lingual artery* (Figs 41.3 & 41.5). Trace it from its commencement in the external carotid till it disappears under the hyoglossus muscle. It may have a common stem of origin with the facial artery and its branches form a major source of blood supply to the tongue. Also look for the occipital artery branching off from the external carotid artery and trace it posteriorly to the back of the head.

In the interval between the thyroid cartilage and the hyoid bone look for the *internal laryngeal nerve* (Fig. 41.3). This is a branch of the *superior laryngeal* branch of the vagus nerve and it gives sensory innervation to the lower part of the pharynx and also to the laryngeal mucosa above the level of the vocal cords. The nerve is accompanied by the *superior laryngeal artery*, a branch of the superior thyroid artery.

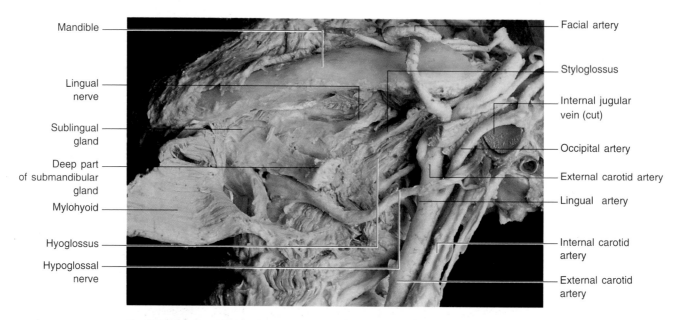

Fig. 41.5 **Structures deep to the mylohyoid muscle**

42

The external aspect of the pharynx

The pharynx is a muscular tube attached to the base of the skull. Below the level of the cricoid cartilage it opens into the oesophagus. For descriptive purposes, the interior of the pharynx is divided into *nasopharynx*, *oropharynx*, and *hypopharynx* or *laryngeal part of the pharynx*. The nasal cavity opens into the nasopharynx, the oropharynx is continuous with the oral cavity and the larynx opens into the hypopharynx. The exterior of the pharynx will be examined here; the interior of the pharynx will be exposed in later dissections.

The wall of the pharynx is made up of mucosa, submucosa, muscles and a thin layer of fascia covering the muscles — the buccopharyngeal fascia (this fascia also covers the buccinator). The circular muscles of the pharynx are the three pharyngeal constrictors (superior, middle and inferior). These are arranged like three paper cups one inside the other. The pharyngeal wall is deficient in front where the pharynx opens into the nasal, oral and laryngeal cavities.

Removal of the vertebral column

This is a dissection designed to reveal the exterior of the pharynx, the carotid sheath, the glossopharyngeal and the vagus nerves and the cervical part of the sympathetic trunk. The dissection requires the removal of the vertebral column which lies behind the pharynx and oesophagus. Follow the instruction given below carefully:

1. find the plane between the pharynx and the vertebrae. Separate it by inserting your hand and then opening your fingers
2. free the carotid sheath and other soft tissue structures from the vertebral column
3. cut down through the muscles posterior to the vertebral column below the skull until you hit the vertebrae, *keeping the cut as close to the skull as possible*. Similarly

cut the muscles lateral to the vertebrae
4. insert a bone chisel or a strong scalpel with a fixed blade and cut through the ligaments between the bones
5. now one person must hold the head very firmly and the other twist the vertebrae back and forth until the vertebral column comes off. If this does not happen, check that you have cut all the muscles and ligaments and try again.

Refer to Figure 42.1 and carefully remove the fascia covering the pharynx and identify the *superior*, *middle* and *inferior constrictor muscles* of the pharynx. Note that they fuse together in the *pharyngeal raphe* in the midline at the back.

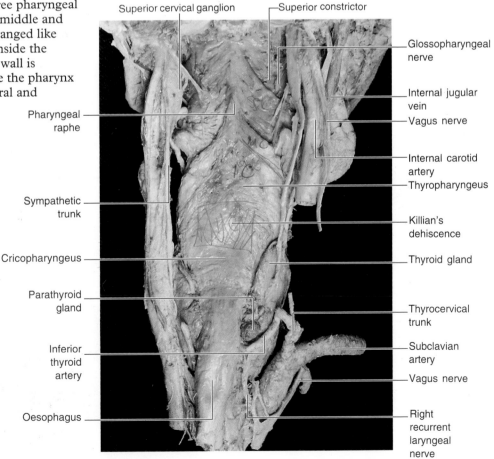

Superior cervical ganglion

Superior constrictor

Glossopharyngeal nerve

Internal jugular vein

Vagus nerve

Internal carotid artery

Thyropharyngeus

Killian's dehiscence

Thyroid gland

Thyrocervical trunk

Subclavian artery

Vagus nerve

Right recurrent laryngeal nerve

Pharyngeal raphe

Sympathetic trunk

Cricopharyngeus

Parathyroid gland

Inferior thyroid artery

Oesophagus

Fig. 42.1 **Pharynx, thyroid gland and the major nerves and vessels of the neck seen from behind**

Constrictor muscles (Fig. 42.2)

The origins of the constrictor muscles are as follows. The superior constrictor takes origin from the *pterygomandibular raphe* which extends from the *medial pterygoid plate* to the mandible; the middle from the *hyoid bone*; and the inferior constrictor from the *thyroid cartilage* (the thyropharyngeus) and the *cricoid cartilage* (the cricopharyngeus). The inner aspect of the constrictors are lined by the thick *pharyngobasilar fascia* which is attached to the *pharyngeal tubercle*, the *auditory (Eustachian) tube* and the *medial pterygoid plate*. This fascia bridges the gap between the superior constrictor and the base of the skull.

Examine the base of the skull and note the points of attachment of the superior constrictor and the pharyngobasilar fascia (Fig. 42.3).

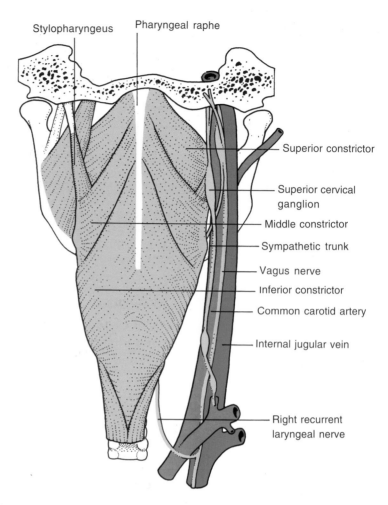

Fig. 42.2 **Pharynx: posterior view.** The right-hand side of the illustration shows related nerves and vessels

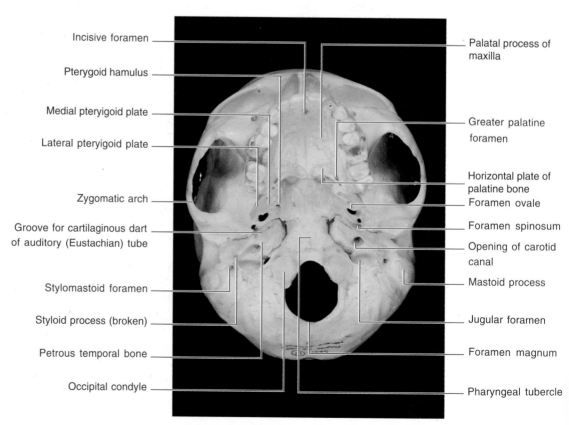

Fig. 42.3 **Base of the skull seen from below**

∗ The weakest part of the pharyngeal wall is in the midline at the back in the lower part of the pharynx. This lies between the diverging fibres of the cricopharyngeal and the thyropharyngeal parts of the inferior constrictor. This area is known as the *Killian's dehiscence* and is the commonest site for a pharyngeal diverticulum (protrusion of the wall due to excessive pressure).

Identify the upper part of the carotid sheath and lateral to that the *styloid process*. Dissect in the interval between the superior and the middle constrictors and expose the *stylopharyngeus* muscle (Fig. 42.1). This takes origin from the styloid process and lies between the external and the internal carotid arteries to reach the interval between the superior and the middle constrictor muscles. Carefully dissect out the *glossopharyngeal nerve* which lies on the surface of the stylopharyngeus.

Glossopharyngeal nerve

The glossopharyngeal nerve (ninth cranial nerve) gives sensory innervation to the posterior third of the tongue and the oropharynx. Its tympanic branch supplies the middle ear and the auditory (Eustachian) tube. It also supplies the stylopharyngeus muscle.

Vagus nerve

The vagus nerve (tenth cranial nerve) is the largest and the most widely distributed of the cranial nerves. It leaves the skull through the jugular foramen and descends through the neck within the carotid sheath. In the neck the vagus gives off the pharyngeal branch, the superior laryngeal nerve and the cardiac branches. The right recurrent laryngeal nerve branches off from the right vagus in the lower part of the neck whereas the left recurrent laryngeal nerve (a branch of the left vagus) is given off in the superior mediastinum.

Clean the *pharyngeal branch of the vagus nerve*. This can be seen breaking up into branches on the pharyngeal wall. Trace it to the vagus between the external and internal carotid arteries.

The pharyngeal branch of the vagus gives motor innervation to the muscles of the pharynx and soft palate. Its fibres originate in the nucleus ambiguus in the brainstem.

Clean the *superior laryngeal branch of the vagus*. It lies deep to the external and the internal carotid arteries.

Superior laryngeal nerve

The superior laryngeal nerve divides into the internal and the external laryngeal nerves. The internal laryngeal nerve has already been examined (p.148). The *external laryngeal nerve* supplies the *cricothyroid muscle* as well as the cricopharyngeal part of the inferior constrictor.

∗ The external laryngeal nerve passes deep to the superior thyroid artery and may be damaged in ligating this vessel. Damage to this causes some weakness of voice due to loss of action of the cricothyroid muscle on the vocal chord.

Identify the *right recurrent laryngeal nerve*. This branches off from the right vagus and winds round the subclavian artery (Fig. 42.1). Trace it from the vagus to the groove between the trachea and the oesophagus and upwards till it disappears under the lower border of the inferior constrictor. Look for the left recurrent laryngeal nerve in the groove between the trachea and the oesophagus on the left side. (This nerve, unlike the one on the right, winds round the ligamentum arteriosum in the thorax, p.52.) Note how closely the two nerves are related to the thyroid gland.

Clean the *inferior thyroid artery* and trace it to the back of the thyroid gland. Note that the inferior thyroid artery crosses the recurrent laryngeal nerve at the lower pole of the thyroid gland (Fig. 42.1).

∗ As the inferior thyroid artery and the recurrent laryngeal nerve are so close to each other near the thyroid gland, in thyroid surgery it is safer to ligate the artery some distance lateral to the gland to avoid damage to the nerve.

Clean the *sympathetic trunk* and identify the large *superior cervical ganglion*.

Cervical sympathetic ganglia

There are three cervical sympathetic ganglia in the neck, the *superior*, *middle* and *inferior ganglia*. The middle cervical ganglion may be absent. The inferior ganglion often fuses with the first thoracic ganglion to form the *stellate ganglion*. The stellate ganglion is situated in front of the neck of the first rib and the transverse process of the seventh cervical vertebra.

∗ Paralysis of the sympathetic trunk at the root of the neck may occur as a result of compression from a tumour in the apex of the lung. This will produce *Horner's syndrome*, characterized by absence of sweating, constriction of the pupil and slight drooping of the eyelid (ptosis). Horner's syndrome can also be caused by a spinal cord lesion at T_1 segment, as well as pressure on the sympathetic trunk by enlarged cervical lymph nodes or an aneurysm of the carotid artery.

43

The larynx

The main function of the larynx is to prevent food and liquid from entering the trachea and lungs. It is also the site of voice production. It is a tube in the midline, above the trachea, and consists of five major cartilages: the *thyroid cartilage*, the *cricoid cartilage*, the two *arytenoid cartilages* and the *epiglottis*. These cartilages are connected by ligaments and muscles. The major cartilages of the larynx are illustrated in Figure 43.1.

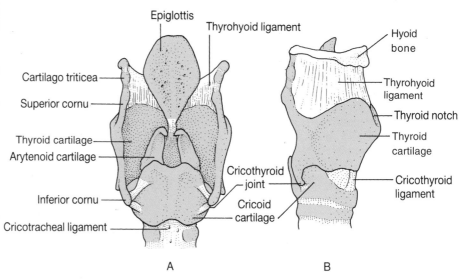

Fig. 43.1 **Cartilages of the larynx and the hyoid bone. A.** Posterior view. **B.** Lateral view

SURFACE ANATOMY
(Fig. 38.1, p.134)

Identify the following on your partner:

- the hyoid bone
- the thyroid cartilage
- the cricoid cartilage
- the tracheal ring below the cricoid cartilage.

Note that the larynx moves up and down with deglutition.

Palpate the gap between the thyroid and the cricoid in the midline. This is occupied by the *cricothyroid ligament* (cricothyroid membrane).

✳ In a dire emergency, where there is obstruction to the upper airway, making an opening in the cricothyroid ligament — *cricothyroid stab* or *laryngotomy* — may be life saving.

Remove the infrahyoid muscles and identify the *cricothyroid muscle* passing between the thyroid and cricoid cartilages (Fig. 43.2).

The cricothyroid muscles tilt the thyroid cartilage downwards on the cricoid and lengthen the vocal cords.

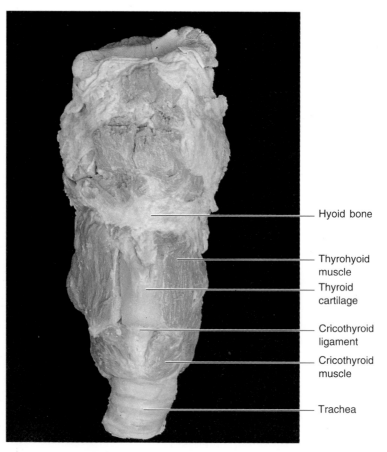

Fig. 43.2 **Larynx: anterior aspect**

Cut the posterior wall of the oesophagus and the pharynx in the midline. Turn the cut ends aside and expose the interior of the pharynx and the posterior aspect of the larynx. Identify the *soft palate* and uvula, the *epiglottis*, the *aryepiglottic folds*, the *inlet of the larynx, posterior aspect of the cricoid* and the *arytenoid* (Figs 43.3 & 43.4). Also note that the larynx is opening into the hypopharynx (laryngeal part of the pharynx) and that a forward extension of the hypopharynx forming a cul de sac by the side of the larynx is the *piriform fossa*.

✳ A malignant tumour arising in the piriform fossa may be 'silent' in the early stages. It may *not* produce difficulty in swallowing, as the space is a recess extending from the main cavity of the pharynx.

During deglutition (swallowing) the inlet of the larynx is closed by elevation of the larynx and approximating it against the back of the tongue. The epiglottis is bent over the inlet. The aryepiglottic folds are approximated. The bolus of food passes through the piriform fossa into the oesophagus. Choking on food is a common cause of laryngeal obstruction and can occur in a person who has had excessive amounts of alcohol.

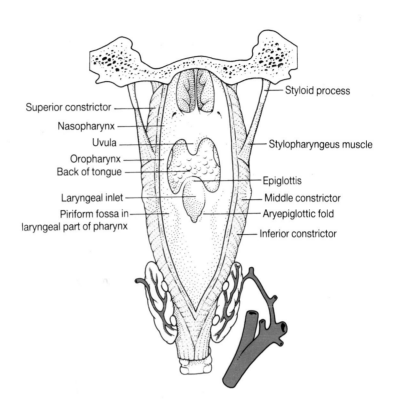

Fig. 43.3 **Pharynx, opened from behind**

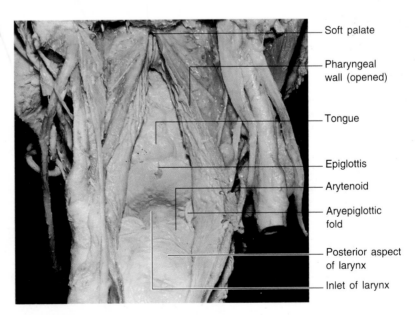

Fig. 43.4 **Pharynx opened from behind showing laryngeal part of pharynx and the laryngeal inlet**

Remove the mucosa from the back of the cricoid and the arytenoids and expose the *posterior cricoarytenoid muscles* (Fig. 43.5). The posterior cricoarytenoids abduct the vocal cords.

Cut vertically along the posterior wall of the trachea and larynx in the midline and open out the larynx.

Identify the vestibular folds and the vocal folds (vocal cords; Fig. 43.6). The space between the vestibular and the vocal folds is the *sinus of the larynx*. The space between the vocal folds is the *rima glottidis*, the narrowest part of the upper airway.

Identify again the *internal laryngeal nerve* (p.148). Note that it pierces the thyrohyoid membrane to enter the piriform fossa in the laryngeal part of the pharynx (Fig. 43.5). This nerve gives sensory innervation to the laryngeal part of the pharynx as well as to the part of the larynx above the vocal cord.

✳ Foreign bodies such as a fish bone may get lodged in the piriform fossa. Instrumentation for removal of this may damage the internal laryngeal nerve.

Identify the *recurrent laryngeal nerve* in the groove between the oesophagus and the trachea and trace it into the laryngeal part of the pharynx. This nerve enters the pharynx crossing the lower border of the inferior constrictor muscle.

The nerve lies in the sub-mucosa and can be anaesthetized by topical application of local anaesthetic agents.

The recurrent laryngeal nerve innervates all the *intrinsic muscles* of the larynx except the cricothyroid. The *cricothyroid* is innervated by the *external laryngeal branch* of the superior laryngeal nerve (p.151). The recurrent laryngeal nerve also gives sensory innervation to the part of the larynx below the level of the vocal cords as well as the trachea (see also p. 137).

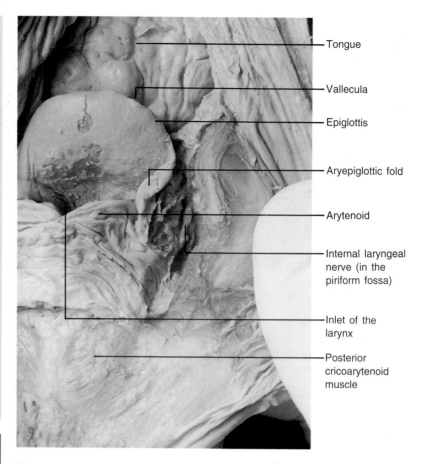

- Tongue
- Vallecula
- Epiglottis
- Aryepiglottic fold
- Arytenoid
- Internal laryngeal nerve (in the piriform fossa)
- Inlet of the larynx
- Posterior cricoarytenoid muscle

Fig. 43.5 **External aspect of the larynx seen from the back** (after partial removal of the mucous membrane)

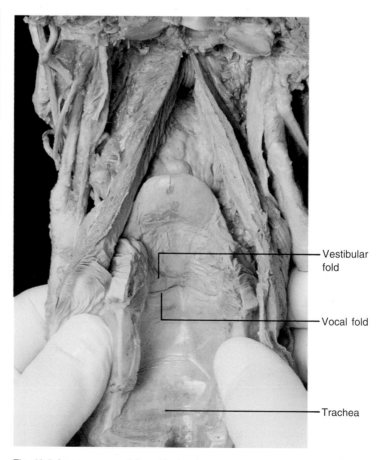

- Vestibular fold
- Vocal fold
- Trachea

Fig. 43.6 **Larynx opened from the back**

✳ The larynx may be viewed in the living by placing a mirror in the oropharynx (Fig. 43.7). The back of the tongue, epiglottis, laryngeal inlet, vestibular folds and the vocal folds can thus be seen. The vestibular folds appear pink, as the blood vessels shine through the mucous membrane. The vocal folds are pale in colour as the mucous membrane is tightly adherent to the underlying connective tissue. When the vocal folds are abducted, the first few tracheal rings can also be seen in the mirror.

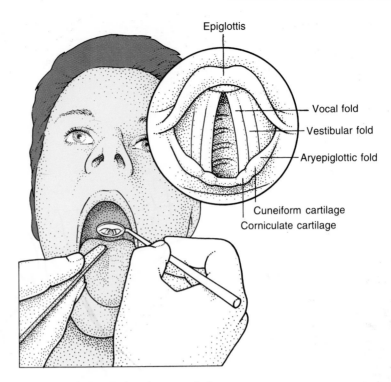

Fig. 43.7 **View of the vocal cords as seen by laryngoscope**

44

The removal of the brain

In this session the brain will be removed so that its surface features can be examined and the cranial cavity studied. To do this the *skull cap (calvarium)* needs to be removed.

Removal of the skull cap

> Make a saw cut around the circumference of the skull at a level 1 cm above the orbital margin and prise out the calvarium using a chisel. Make sure that you do not damage the brain surface while doing this. Remove the calvarium by cutting the *falx cerebri* which is attached to it in the midline.

Study the internal surface of the calvarium (Fig. 44.1). Identify the *superior sagittal sinus* along the upper border of the falx cerebri. The *falx cerebri* is the vertical extension of the inner layer of *dura mater* and it lies between the two *cerebral hemispheres* (Fig. 44.2). The outer layer of dura mater is the inner periosteum of the skull bones. The *inferior sagittal sinus* lies along the lower free border of the falx cerebri (Fig. 44.3).

Examine the cut surface of the bone. Note the inner and outer plates of compact bone and the intervening spongy bone.

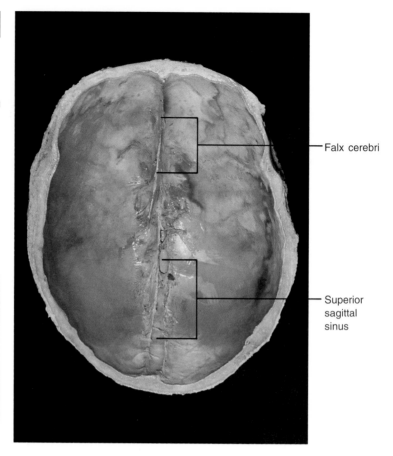

Fig. 44.1 **Interior of the calvarium**

— Falx cerebri

— Superior sagittal sinus

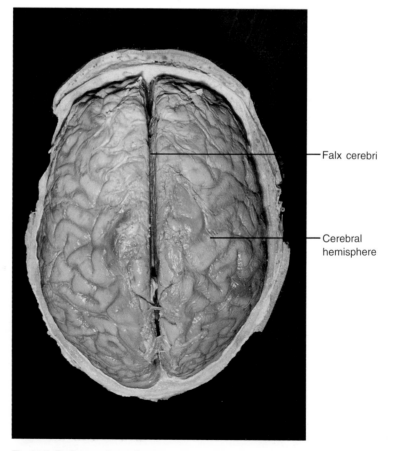

Fig. 44.2 **Brain seen from above**

— Falx cerebri

— Cerebral hemisphere

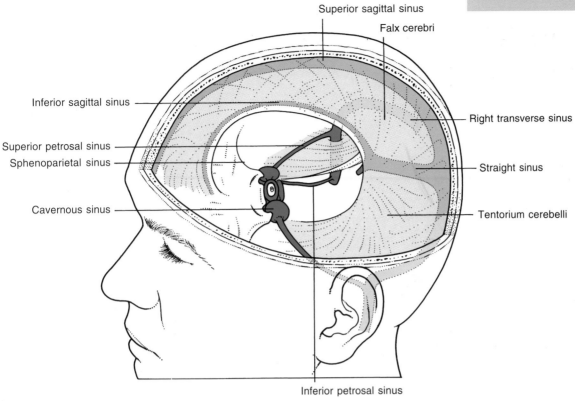

Superior sagittal sinus

Falx cerebri

Inferior sagittal sinus

Right transverse sinus

Superior petrosal sinus

Sphenoparietal sinus

Straight sinus

Cavernous sinus

Tentorium cerebelli

Inferior petrosal sinus

Fig. 44.3 **Venous sinuses**

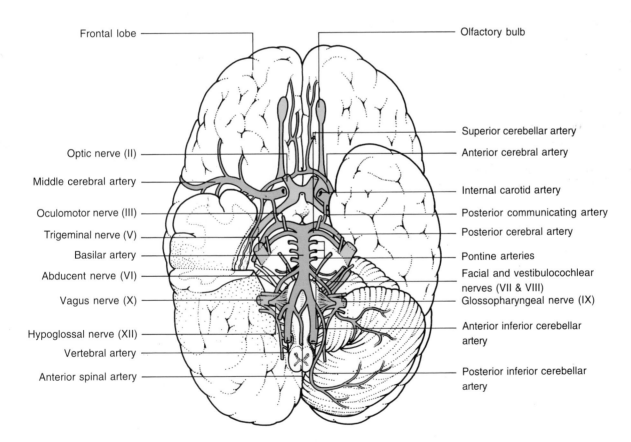

Frontal lobe

Olfactory bulb

Optic nerve (II)

Superior cerebellar artery

Anterior cerebral artery

Middle cerebral artery

Internal carotid artery

Oculomotor nerve (III)

Posterior communicating artery

Trigeminal nerve (V)

Posterior cerebral artery

Basilar artery

Pontine arteries

Abducent nerve (VI)

Facial and vestibulocochlear nerves (VII & VIII)

Vagus nerve (X)

Glossopharyngeal nerve (IX)

Hypoglossal nerve (XII)

Anterior inferior cerebellar artery

Vertebral artery

Anterior spinal artery

Posterior inferior cerebellar artery

Fig. 44.4 **Inferior surface of the brain.** The cerebellar hemisphere and part of the temporal lobe have been removed on the right side

Removal of the brain

First study Figures 44.4 & 44.5 to become familiar with the structures you will come across during this dissection.

Lift the frontal lobes of the hemispheres and identify the *olfactory bulbs* lying on the cribriform fossa. Detach these from the bone and raise the hemispheres further. The *optic nerves* and the *internal carotid arteries* will come into view; cut these. Behind these structures identify the *oculomotor nerve* and the *trochlear nerve* and cut them. Disentangle the temporal lobes from the middle cranial fossa and gently pull the brain backwards. The *abducens nerves* will now be visible on either side of the midline. Sever them. The two *cerebral peduncles* will come into view. Lateral to these the *trigeminal nerves* will be seen piercing the dura mater. Cut the nerve on each side. Now feel the line of attachment of the *tentorium cerebelli* along the upper border of the petrous temporal bone (Fig. 44.5). Cut the tentorium cerebelli along its attachment to the bone. Make sure that this is done on both sides and that the cut is complete. The tentorium cerebelli roofs the *posterior cranial fossa* and it lies between the *cerebellum* and the cerebral hemispheres. Once the tentorium cerebelli is severed from its attachments you should be able to insert your fingers into the posterior cranial fossa and feel the lower part of the brainstem (*medulla oblongata*). Cut the medulla as low as possible and gently lift up the brain As you do so, incise the remaining cranial nerves and the vertebral arteries in the posterior cranial fossa.

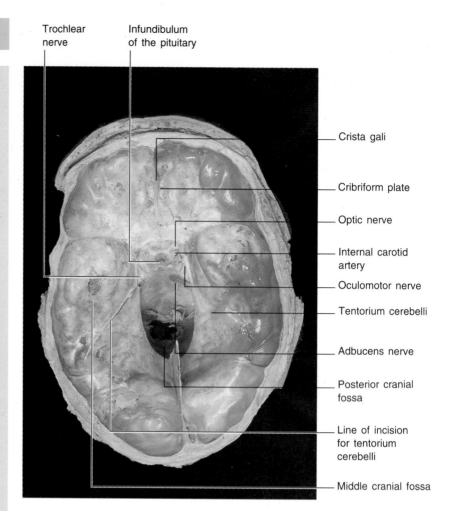

Fig. 44.5 **Cranial cavity**

Gross examination of the brain

Identify the major parts of the brain: the two cerebral hemispheres, the brainstem and the cerebellum. The brainstem is formed from above downwards by the *midbrain*, the *pons* and the medulla oblongata. On the inferior surface of the brain identify the cranial nerves and also the major arteries of the brain contributing to the *circle of Willis* (Fig. 44.6).

The brain is covered by the three meninges: the dura mater, the *arachnoid mater* and the *pia mater*. The space between the arachnoid and the pia is the *subarachnoid space* which contains the *cerebrospinal fluid* (*CSF*). It also contains the major blood vessels of the brain, including the circle of Willis.

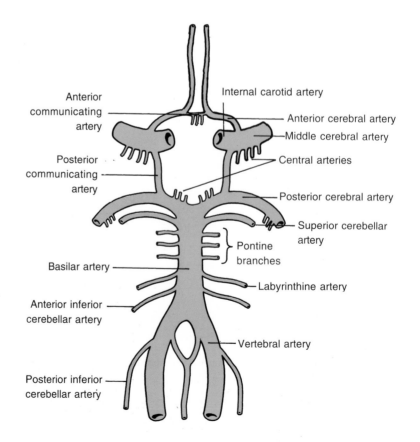

Fig. 44.6 **Circle of Willis.** The central arteries supply the corpus striatum, internal capsule, diencephalon and midbrain

45

The cranial fossae and dural venous sinuses

In this session the structures seen in the cranial cavity after removal of the brain will be examined.

Refer to Figure 45.1 and examine a dry skull and study the osteology of the three cranial fossae.

Refer to Figures 45.2 and 45.3 and identify the structures described in the following paragraphs on your specimen.

Examine the *anterior cranial fossa.* The falx cerebri is attached to the crista galli. The *cribriform plate* of the ethmoid transmits the *olfactory nerves.*

> ✳ The cribriform plate forms the roof of the nose. Tumours from the upper part of the nasal cavity can spread into the anterior cranial fossa. Fractures of the anterior cranial fossa may produce bleeding and leakage of cerebrospinal fluid (CSF) through the nasal cavity.

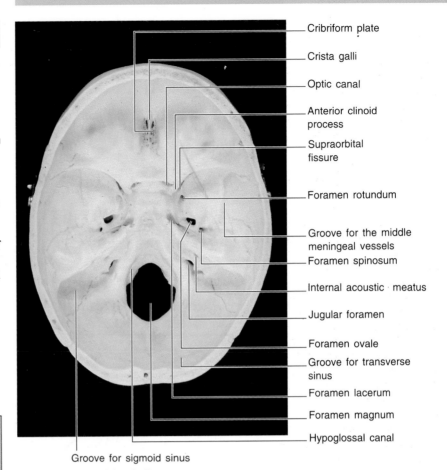

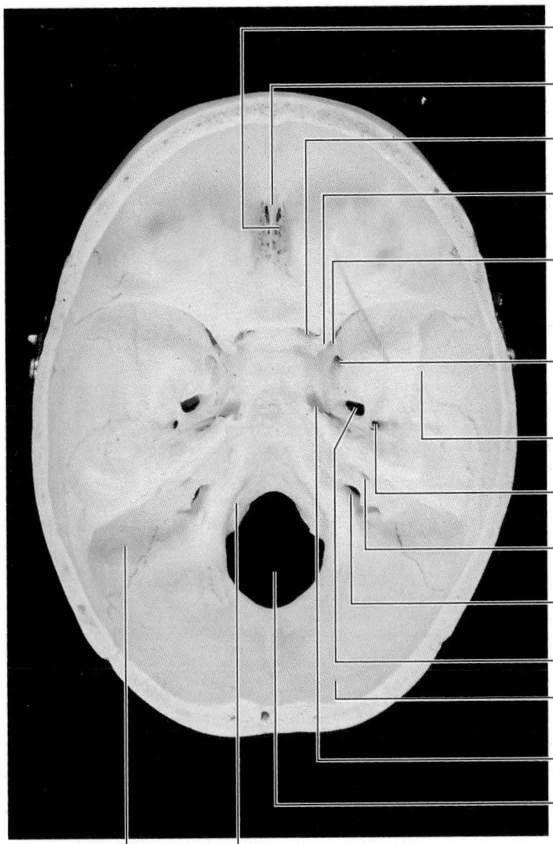
Cribriform plate
Crista galli
Optic canal
Anterior clinoid process
Supraorbital fissure
Foramen rotundum
Groove for the middle meningeal vessels
Foramen spinosum
Internal acoustic meatus
Jugular foramen
Foramen ovale
Groove for transverse sinus
Foramen lacerum
Foramen magnum
Hypoglossal canal
Groove for sigmoid sinus

Fig. 45.1 **Interior of the skull**

Identify the *optic nerve* and the *ophthalmic artery* passing through the *optic canal.*

In the middle of the *middle cranial fossa* is the *sella turcica* (hypophyseal fossa) containing the pituitary gland. The sella turcica is roofed by a fold of dura mater, the *diaphragma sellae* and this is pierced by the infundibulum. The diaphragma sellae is attached to the *anterior* and *posterior clinoid processes.*

> Remove the diaphragma sellae and expose the pituitary gland.

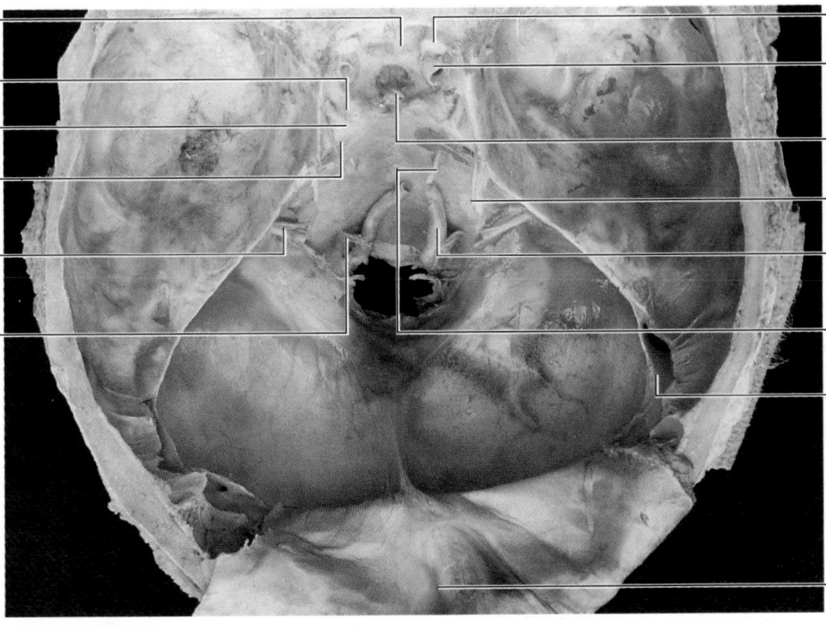
Diaphragma sellae
Oculomotor nerve
Cavernous sinus
Trochlear nerve
Facial and vestibulocochlear nerve
Hypoglossal nerve
Optic nerve
Internal carotid artery
Infundibulum
Trigeminal nerve
Vertebral artery
Abducens nerve
Transverse sinus
Tentorium cerebelli

Fig. 45.2 **Middle and posterior cranial fossae**

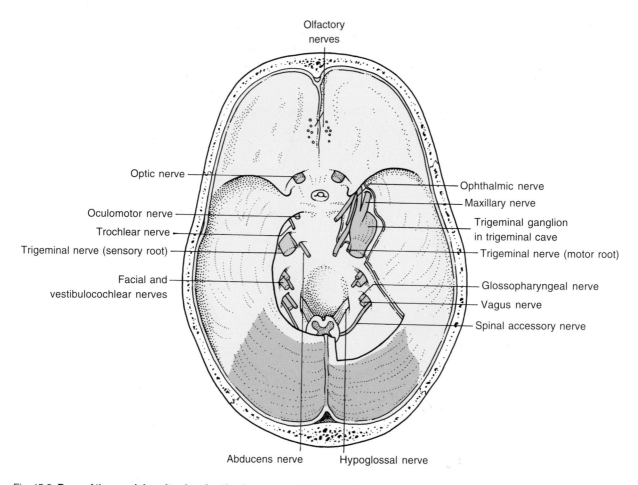

Fig. 45.3 **Base of the cranial cavity showing the dura mater and the cranial nerves.** On the right side, part of the tentorium cerebelli and the roof of the trigeminal cave have been removed

Lateral to the pituitary gland, the dura mater contains the *cavernous sinuses,* one on either side. A number of cranial nerves and the internal carotid artery pass through the cavernous sinus. These are illustrated in Figure 45.4.

✳ Infection can reach the cavernous sinus from the face and the eye because of its venous connections. These connections are shown in Figure 45.5.

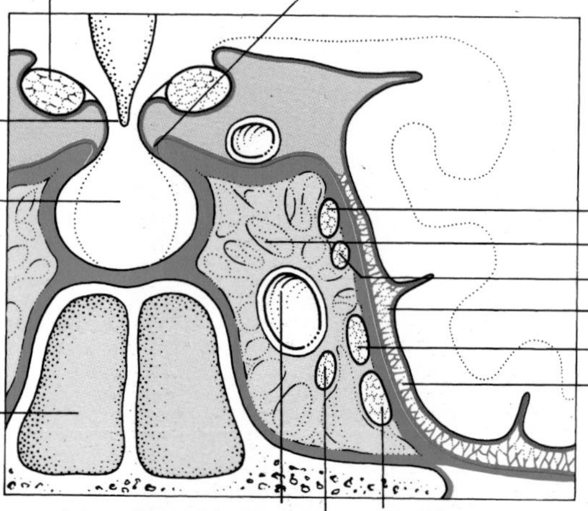

Carefully incise the dura mater of the cavernous sinus and expose the structures in it (Fig. 45.4). Note that the carotid artery is S-shaped when it is inside the sinus.

Identify the *trigeminal nerve* as it enters the middle cranial fossa. It takes a prolongation of the dura from the posterior cranial fossa with it (*trigeminal cave or Meckel's cave*).

Incise the dura over the trigeminal nerve and expose the *trigeminal ganglion* in the Meckel's cave in the middle cranial fossa (Fig. 45.3). Trace the three divisions of the nerve forward till they leave the skull. The *ophthalmic division* goes through the *supraorbital fissure*, the *maxillary* through the *foramen rotundum* and the *mandibular division* through the *foramen ovale.*

Fig. 45.4 **Cavernous sinus**

Note the groove for the *middle meningeal artery* and *vein* on the inner aspect of the skull (Figure 45.1). The middle meningeal artery enters the skull through the *foramen spinosum*. The middle meningeal artery and vein can rupture in head injury and produce an *extradural haemorrhage*.

Cut around the margins of the tentorium cerebelli and remove it. This will expose the *transverse and sigmoid sinuses* as well as the two *petrosal sinuses*. Note the connections of these sinuses by referring to Figure 44.3, p.157 and compare this to Figure 45.6 which is an angiogram taken in the venous phase.

Refer to Figs 45.2 and 45.3 and identify the cut ends of *the facial (VII)* and *vestibulocochlear (VIII) nerves* as they enter the *internal acoustic (auditory) meatus*. Find the *glossopharyngeal (IX), vagus (X)* and the *accessory (XI) nerves* entering the *jugular foramen*. Note that the sigmoid sinus and the inferior petrosal sinus also leave the skull through this foramen. Identify the spinal part of the accessory nerve coming up through the *foramen magnum* and going into the jugular foramen. Also identify the two vertebral arteries coming through the foramen magnum. Lastly trace the *hypoglossal nerve (XII)* into the hypoglossal canal.

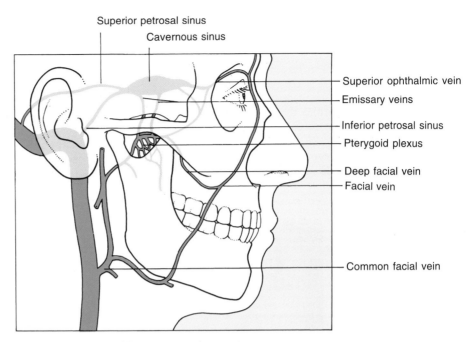

Fig. 45.5 **Connections of the cavernous sinus**

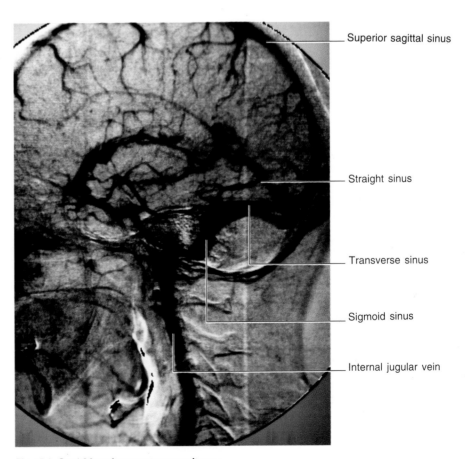

Fig. 45.6 **Carotid angiogram: venous phase**

46

The orbit

The orbit which contains the eyeball and the structures surrounding it will now be dissected. These structures include the extraocular muscles and their nerves as well as the optic nerves and the branches of the ophthalmic division of the trigeminal nerve. The orbit also contains the ophthalmic artery, which supplies the eye, and the corresponding orbital veins.

OSTEOLOGY

Refer to Figure 46.1 and study the bones forming the walls of the orbit using a dry skull.

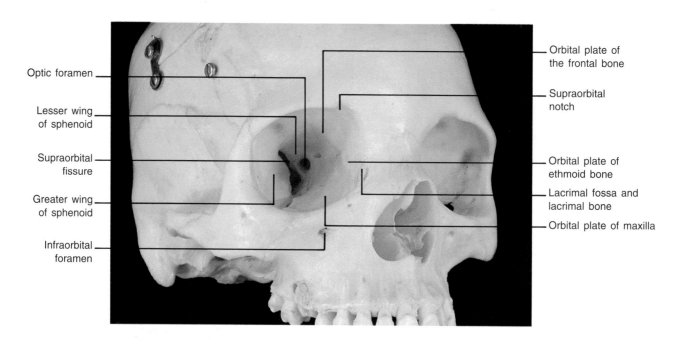

Optic foramen

Lesser wing of sphenoid

Supraorbital fissure

Greater wing of sphenoid

Infraorbital foramen

Orbital plate of the frontal bone

Supraorbital notch

Orbital plate of ethmoid bone

Lacrimal fossa and lacrimal bone

Orbital plate of maxilla

Fig. 46.1 **Bones forming the walls of the orbit**

Remove the periosteum from the anterior cranial fossa and expose the *orbital plate* of the *frontal bone* and the *lesser wing* of the *sphenoid* forming the roof of the orbit. Remove this by making saw cuts on the medial and lateral borders of the roof and carefully nibbling away the bone using a bone forceps. You should do this by keeping the inner periosteum of the roof intact.

Carefully remove the periosteum and expose the *frontal, lacrimal* and the *trochlear nerves* (Fig. 46.2). The trochlear will be seen entering the superior oblique muscle. Clean the muscle. The frontal nerve will be lying on the levator palpebrae superioris muscle. Clean the muscle and the supratrochlear and the supraorbital branches of the frontal nerve.

The frontal and the lacrimal nerves, along with the nasociliary nerve, are terminal branches of the ophthalmic division of the trigeminal nerve. These branches are given off in the cavernous sinus. The frontal nerve, through its two branches, supplies the skin of the forehead and scalp and the frontal air sinus. The lacrimal nerve supplies the lacrimal gland, the upper eyelid and the conjunctiva.

Levator palpebrae superioris is inserted into the upper eyelid. Its main innervation is by the *oculomotor nerve,* but a few of the deeper fibres are supplied by *sympathetic nerves.*

✳ Paralysis of the oculomotor nerve will produce *drooping of the eyelid (ptosis).* This can also result as a consequence of sympathetic trunk paralysis in the neck.

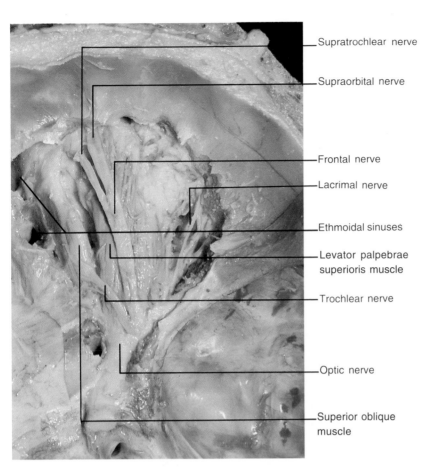

Fig. 46.2 **Structures of the orbit seen after removal of its roof**

Lift up the levator palpebrae superioris and note its nerve supply entering the muscle through the underlying superior rectus. Remove the frontal nerve and the levator palpebrae superioris and expose the superior rectus muscle (Fig. 46.3). Clean this and note its attachment to the upper surface of the sclera. Also clean the superior oblique. Its tendon winds round a fibrous 'pulley' (trochlea) at the medial angle of the orbit. The tendon then spreads out to be inserted into the posterolateral quadrant of the eyeball.

All the eye movements refer to movements of the front of the eye. The *superior rectus* deviates the front of the eye upwards and medially. The *superior oblique* deviates the eye downwards and laterally as it pulls its insertion towards the trochlea. This muscle is supplied by the *trochlear nerve*.

The combined action of the superior oblique and the inferior rectus is essential for looking straight downwards

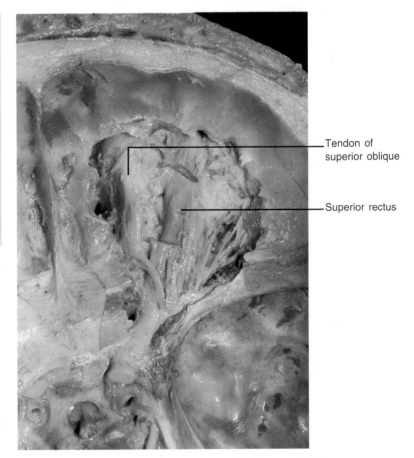

Fig. 46.3 **Orbit after removal of part of levator palpebrae superioris**

* If the trochlear nerve is paralysed, when the patient looks downwards the paralysed eye will point downwards and medially by the action of inferior rectus on its own. This will result in *double vision (diplopia)* in going down stairs.

Remove the superior rectus and the belly of the superior oblique. Trace the tendon off the superior oblique to its insertion. Refer to Figure 46.4 and clean the optic nerve, ophthalmic artery, nasociliary nerve (branch of the ophthalmic nerve) and the medial and lateral rectus muscles. *The optic nerve throughout its course is lined by the three layers of meninges.* Cerebrospinal fluid (CSF) circulates in the subarachnoid space around the optic nerve. Look for the abducens nerve entering the inner surface of the lateral rectus.

* The *lateral rectus* deviates the eye laterally. Paralysis of the abducens nerve will produce diplopia when looking towards the paralysed side.

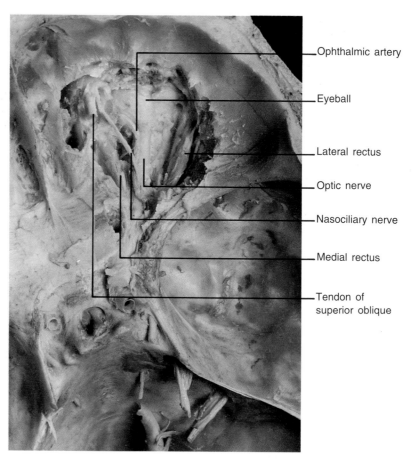

Ophthalmic artery

Eyeball

Lateral rectus

Optic nerve

Nasociliary nerve

Medial rectus

Tendon of superior oblique

Fig. 46.4 **Orbit after removal of superior rectus and superior oblique**

Medial rectus deviates the eye medially and is supplied by the oculomotor nerve.

The *nasociliary nerve* gives sensory innervation to the eye. It supplies the eye through the *long* and *short ciliary nerves* which enter the back of the eyeball. The short ciliary nerves come as branches of the *ciliary ganglion* which is connected to the nasociliary nerve. Parasympathetic fibres carried by the oculomotor nerve synapse in the ganglion and reach the eye through the short ciliary nerves. The parasympathetic fibres supply the *ciliary muscles* and the *constrictor pupillae* in the eye. Besides sensory fibres, the long ciliary nerves carry sympathetic fibres to the eye. These supply the blood vessels and the *dilator pupillae* muscle.

The nasociliary nerve also supplies the ethmoidal sinuses through the *anterior* and *posterior ethmoidal nerves*. The anterior ethmoidal nerve is long and it also innervates the nasal cavity and the skin of the nose.

After giving off the branches described above, the nasociliary nerve terminates near the medial angle of the eye as the *infratrochlear nerve* which supplies the medial part of the upper eyelid and the corresponding conjunctiva.

Remove the optic nerve and expose the inferior rectus, which lies below it parallel to the superior rectus. Note its insertion to the undersurface of the eyeball. Cut this and lift the eye upwards and clean the inferior oblique on the floor of the orbit. The muscle passes from the medial part of the orbit posterolaterally to be inserted onto the posterolateral quadrant of the eyeball.

The *inferior rectus* moves the eye downwards and medially and the *inferior oblique* deviates it upwards and laterally. Both are supplied by the oculomotor nerve.

* *Oculomotor nerve paralysis* will paralyse all the extraocular muscles except the lateral rectus (abducens nerve) and the superior oblique (trochlear nerve). It will also paralyse the levator palpebral superioris resulting in ptosis and the paralysis of the constrictor pupillae producing dilatation of the pupil.

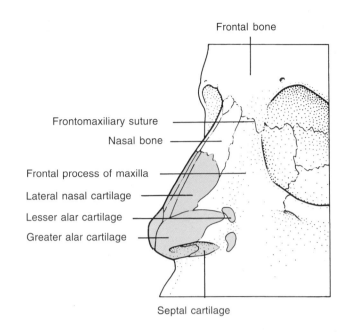

Fig. 47.1 **Cartilages and bones of the external nose**

47

The nasal cavity and paranasal sinuses

The remaining dissections are better done on a bisected head.

SURFACE ANATOMY

Examine the *external nose* noting its bony and cartilaginous parts (Fig. 47.1). Also examine the antero-inferior part of the *nasal septum*; this part of the septum is cartilaginous and is mobile.

> ✳ Fractures of the nose are extremely common, often due to a direct blow during fights.

Each nasal cavity has a roof, floor, lateral wall and a medial wall formed by the nasal septum. It is pyramidal in shape with a narrow upper part and slightly wider base. The *roof* is formed by the *cribriform plate of the ethmoid* and the *body of the sphenoid*. The *hard palate* forms the *floor*.

The *nasal septum* has a bony and a cartilaginous part. In the upper part it is formed by the *perpendicular plate* of the ethmoid bone and behind and below by the *vomer*, a single midline bone. The gap in front, between these two bones, is bridged by the *septal cartilage*.

> ✳ The septum may often be deflected to one side. This condition may cause nasal obstruction and headache.

Examine the nasal septum and identify the part formed by the vomer and the perpendicular plate of the ethmoid. Anteriorly is the septal cartilage. Note that a thick mucoperiosteum covers the septum (Fig. 47.2). Remove the septum and examine the lateral wall of the nasal cavity.

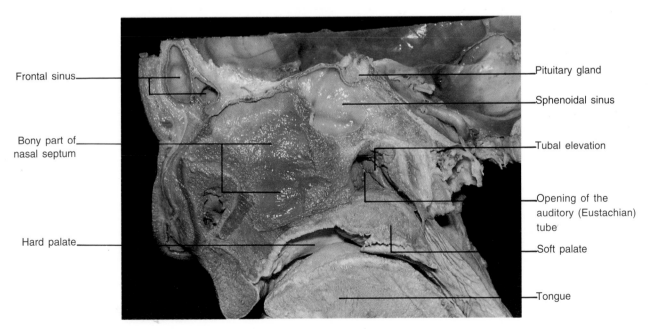

Fig. 47.2 **Nasal septum, nasopharynx, palate and tongue**

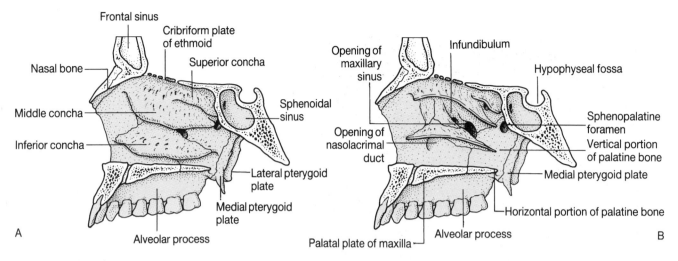

Fig. 47.3 **Bony lateral wall of the nasal cavity. A.** Bones complete. **B.** After partial removal of the conchae

Examine the lateral wall on a bisected skull. The lateral wall is formed by the maxilla. Here the opening of the maxillary sinus is overlapped by the ethmoid, the lacrimal bone, the perpendicular plate of the palatine bone and the inferior concha. Projecting from the lateral wall are the *superior, middle and inferior conchae* dividing the nasal cavity into the *superior, middle and inferior meatuses.* Each meatus is seen below the respective concha. The inferior concha is the largest and is a separate bone. The other two are parts of the ethmoid bone.

∗ The *inferior meatus* is the widest part of the nasal cavity. Nasal intubations are done through this region. Hypertrophy of the inferior concha may produce difficulty in such intubation.

Refer to Figure 47.3 and identify the three conchae and the meatuses. The space above and behind the superior meatus is the *sphenoethmoidal recess.* Remove the inferior concha, peel off the mucosa in the inferior meatus and define the *nasolacrimal duct.* The duct extending from the lacrimal sac drains the lacrimal fluid from the conjunctival sac.

Remove the middle concha and expose the *hiatus semilunaris* (Fig. 47.4). This receives the openings of the *frontal, anterior ethmoidal* and *maxillary sinuses* (Fig. 47.5).

The maxillary sinus (antrum of Highmore) has the opening in the upper part of its medial wall. Hence the sinus may drain inefficiently. The sinus inferiorly is related to the upper premolar and molar teeth. The maxillary sinus can be infected from the nasal cavity or from caries of the upper teeth.

The infraorbital nerve enclosed in a canal, passes through the maxillary sinus.

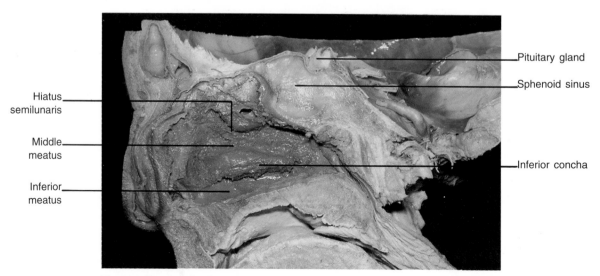

Fig. 47.4 **Nasal cavity after removal of the middle concha**

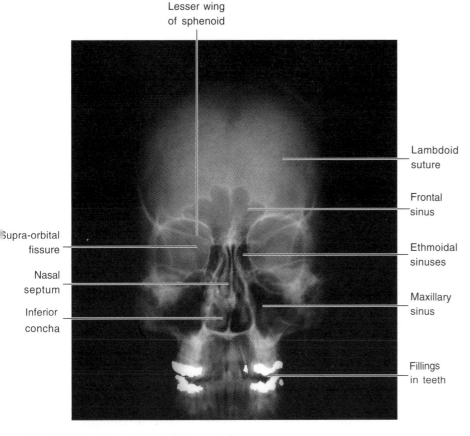

Lesser wing of sphenoid

Lambdoid suture

Frontal sinus

Ethmoidal sinuses

Maxillary sinus

Supra-orbital fissure

Nasal septum

Inferior concha

Fillings in teeth

Fig. 47.5 **PA radiograph of the paranasal sinuses**

The radiological appearance of the paranasal sinuses is shown in Figure 47.5.

> * Malignant tumours in the upper part of the nasal cavity, which are often silent in the early stages, can spread into the cranial cavity through the cribriform plate of the ethmoid. They can also spread into the orbit.

The nerves and vessels of the nasal cavity are shown in Figure 47.6. The innervation is by branches of the *maxillary* and *ophthalmic nerves*. The arterial supply comes from branches of the *external* and *internal carotid arteries*.

The *posterior ethmoidal sinus* opens into the superior meatus and the *sphenoidal sinus* into the *sphenoethmoidal recess*. Note that the pituitary fossa lies above the sphenoidal sinus which is also closely related to the cavernous sinus and the internal carotid artery.

> * The close proximity of the openings of the paranasal sinuses in the middle meatus can aid in the spread of infection from one sinus to another.

> * Surgical access to the pituitary gland is often through the nasal cavity and the sphenoid sinus.

> * Bleeding from the nasal cavity *(epistaxis)* is common. The commonest site is *'Little's area'*, in the antero-inferior part of the septum, where many vessels anastomose.

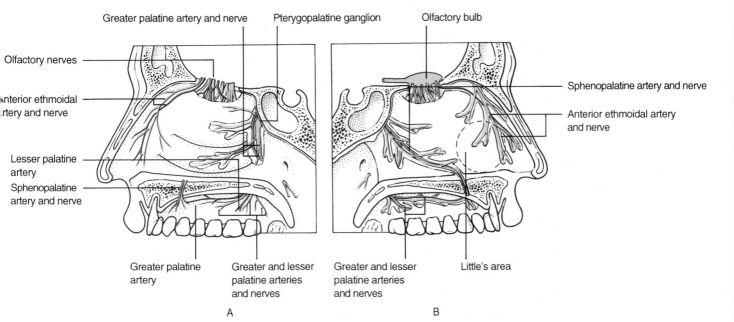

Greater palatine artery and nerve

Pterygopalatine ganglion

Olfactory bulb

Olfactory nerves

Anterior ethmoidal artery and nerve

Lesser palatine artery

Sphenopalatine artery and nerve

Sphenopalatine artery and nerve

Anterior ethmoidal artery and nerve

Greater palatine artery

Greater and lesser palatine arteries and nerves

Greater and lesser palatine arteries and nerves

Little's area

A

B

Fig. 47.6 **Arteries and nerves of the nasal cavity. A.** Lateral wall. **B.** Nasal septum

48

The oral cavity, oropharynx, soft palate and nasopharynx

Very little dissection is necessary during this session. The anatomy of the oral cavity is better learned by examination of the living!

Oral cavity

Examine your partner's mouth, refer to Figure 48.1 and study the features of the tongue. The velvety appearance of the dorsum of the tongue is produced by projections known as papillae. The pointed ones are the *filiform papillae*, which outnumber the reddish and more rounded *fungiform papillae*. Towards the back of the tongue identify the large *vallate papillae*. Just behind the vallate papillae there is a V-shaped *sulcus terminalis* with the apex of the V directed backwards. At the apex is the *foramen caecum* from which the *thyroglossal duct*, which gave rise to the thyroid gland, developed. Behind the sulcus there is a collection of lymphoid tissue forming the *lingual tonsil*.

Lift up the tongue and examine the floor of the mouth and identify the *frenulum* and the *openings of the submandibular ducts* (Fig. 48.1B).

The tongue is a collection of striated muscle which is divided into an *intrinsic* and an *extrinsic* group.

The intrinsic group consists of *transverse, longitudinal and vertical* muscle groups and these change the shape of the tongue. The extrinsic muscles attach the tongue to the adjoining structures. The muscles on each side are the *hyoglossus, palatoglossus, genioglossus and styloglossus* (Fig. 48.2). These muscles move the tongue during mastication, swallowing and speech. All the muscles of the tongue, except the palatoglossus, are supplied by the *hypoglossal nerve*. The innervation of the palatoglossus is by the vagus nerve, through its pharyngeal branch.

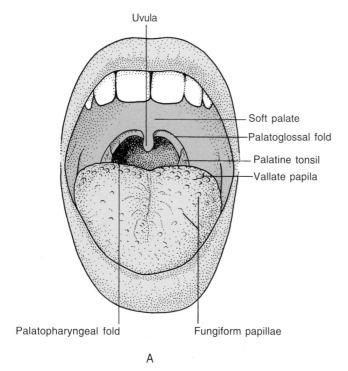

Uvula

Soft palate
Palatoglossal fold
Palatine tonsil
Vallate papila

Palatopharyngeal fold   Fungiform papillae

A

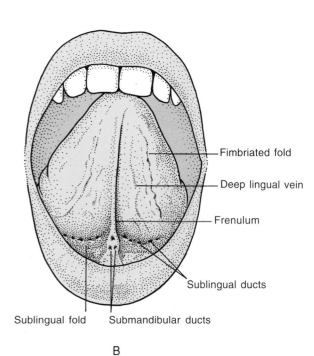

Fimbriated fold

Deep lingual vein

Frenulum

Sublingual ducts

Sublingual fold   Submandibular ducts

B

Fig. 48.1 **Buccal cavity. A.** Mouth and oropharynx. **B.** Inferior surface of the tongue and the floor of the mouth

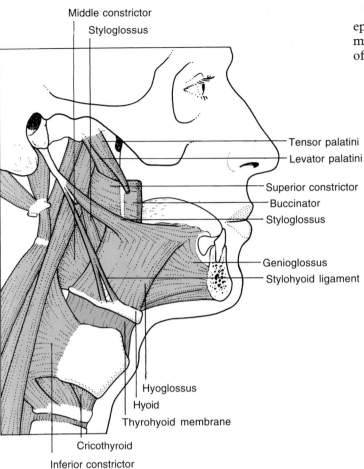

Fig. 48.2 **Muscles of the tongue and pharynx**

Labels in figure:
Middle constrictor
Styloglossus
Tensor palatini
Levator palatini
Superior constrictor
Buccinator
Styloglossus
Genioglossus
Stylohyoid ligament
Hyoglossus
Hyoid
Thyrohyoid membrane
Cricothyroid
Inferior constrictor

The valleculae are seen between the tongue and the epiglottis as depressions one on either side of the midline. The valleculae are common sites for impaction of fish bones.

The sensory innervation of the tongue is shown in Figure 48.3. The anterior two-thirds is supplied by the *lingual nerve* and the posterior third by the *glossopharyngeal*. Taste sensation from the anterior two-thirds is through the *chorda tympani nerve* and from the posterior third through the glossopharyngeal.

Oropharynx

Examine the oropharynx. This contains the *palatine tonsil* commonly known as the 'tonsil' (Fig. 48.1A). The tonsil atrophies in old age and may not be present in dissection-room specimens. Examine your partner's throat and you may be able to identify the tonsil if it has not been surgically removed (tonsillectomy).

The *palatoglossal* and *palatopharyngeal* folds bound the *tonsillar fossa*. These are produced by the palatoglossal and palatopharyngeal muscles. The tonsillar bed is formed by the superior constrictor muscle. The main sensory innervation of the oropharynx is through the *glossopharyngeal nerve*.

* The tonsil has a rich blood supply. The *tonsillar branch of the facial artery* enters it through the superior constrictor. The *paratonsillar vein,* lying deep to the tonsil, is a usual source of bleeding during tonsillectomy.

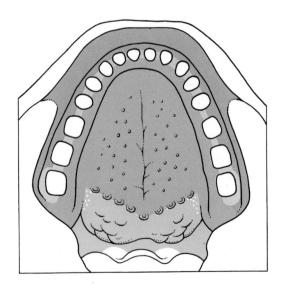

Fig. 48.3 **Sensory nerve supply of the tongue, lower lip and cheek.**
Green = lingual nerve; red = glossopharyngeal nerve; brown = buccal nerve; blue = mental nerve; yellow = inferior alveolar nerve

Palate

The roof of the mouth is the palate. The anterior two-thirds is bony, forming the *hard palate* and the posterior third, the *soft palate*, is muscular.

Examine the palate in the living. Note the midline projection of the soft palate backwards. This is the uvula. If the subject says 'aah' the soft palate will move upwards. The palatine process of the maxilla and the horizontal plate of the palatine bones forming the hard palate, is shown in Figure 42.3, page 150.

The tensor palatini, the levator palatini, the musculus uvuli, the palatoglossus and the palatopharyngeus form the soft palate.

The *tensor palatini* (Fig. 48.2) takes origin from the base of the skull outside the pharyngeal wall and winds round the *pterygoid hamulus* of the medial pterygoid plate (Fig. 42.3, p.150) to enter the cavity of the pharynx. The tendon spreads out to become the *palatine aponeurosis* to be attached to the posterior aspect of the hard palate. The *levator palatini* takes origin from the base of the skull inside the pharynx and is inserted into the palatine aponeurosis.

Both the tensor and the levator palatini in their upper part are attached to the cartilaginous part of the *Eustachian (auditory) tube*. Their contraction opens the tube to transmit air from the pharynx to the middle ear.

✳ Children with *cleft palate* may develop deafness as this mechanism is often affected.

Note the opening of the Eustachian tube in the nasopharynx (Fig. 47.2, p.165). Remove the mucosa in front of the tube and expose the levator palatini muscle; similarly dissect behind the tube to expose the tensor palatini.

The *palatoglossus muscle* is attached to the tongue and the *palatopharyngeus* merges with the wall of the oropharynx. These two, as mentioned earlier, form the boundaries of the tonsillar fossa. The *musculus uvuli* lies on either side of the midline in the substance of the soft palate.

Nasopharynx

Finally examine the *nasopharynx*. This is the part of the pharynx behind the nasal cavity. It has the opening of the Eustachian tube and, in a younger person, the *nasopharyngeal tonsil* or the *adenoids*. The opening of the Eustachian tube can be identified in the living by looking for the prominent *tubal elevation* (Fig. 47.2, p.165). The tubal opening is in front of the elevation. The *salpingopharyngeal fold*, produced by the muscle of the same name, extends downwards from the tubal elevation.

✳ The Eustachian tube can be blocked by enlargement of the adenoids in throat infections. This condition is common in children. Infection from here can spread into the middle ear through the tube. An early sign of a malignant tumour in the nasopharynx may be deafness due to blockage of the auditory tube. The tumour can also spread through the pharyngeal wall into the branches of the trigeminal nerve which are lying just outside the nasopharynx.

49

The eye and the ear

EYE

Examine the eye in the living. The space between the upper and the lower eyelids is the *palpebral fissure*. The inner surface of the eyelid and the anterior aspect of the sclera are lined by the conjunctiva, and the space between the eyelids and the front of the eyeball is the *conjunctival sac*. The upper and lower limits of the conjunctival sac are called the superior and inferior fornices.

Examine the eyelids. Identify the *lacrimal punctum* on each eyelid (Fig. 49.1). The lacrimal puncta are the openings of the *lacrimal canaliculi* which in turn are connected to the *lacrimal sac* (Fig. 49.2). Note that the upper and lower eyelids meet at either end forming the *medial canthus* and the *lateral canthus* (Fig. 49.1). The red elevation on the medial canthus is the *lacrimal caruncle* and the triangular fold extending from it laterally is the *plica semilunaris*.

Dissection of the eye

Remove the skin from the upper eyelid and expose the fibres of the *palpebral part* of the *orbicularis oculi* muscle.

Contraction of the orbicularis oculi closes the palpebral fissure (blinking). This action also moves the lacrimal fluid (tears) from lateral to medial, thus bathing the cornea.

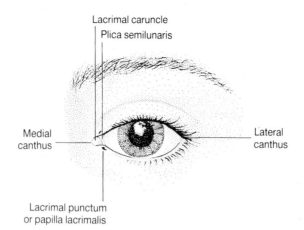

Fig. 49.1 **Eyelids and the eye: anterior view**

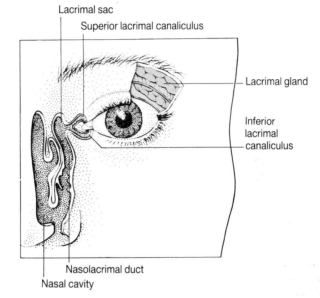

Fig. 49.2 **Lacrimal apparatus**

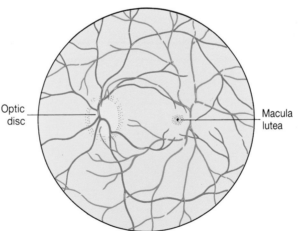

Fig. 49.3 **Retina as seen by ophthalmoscopy**

Remove the fibres of the orbicularis oculi and expose the *lacrimal gland* in the lateral part of the upper eyelid (Fig. 49.2). This is the palpebral part of the gland. Note that the gland also extends into the orbit as its orbital part.

Deep to the orbicularis oculi define the *tarsal plate*, which is the dense fibrous tissue forming the core of the eyelid. The tarsal plates of the two eyelids meet medially and laterally forming the medial and lateral palpebral ligaments,

respectively. Define the *medial palpebral ligament*. Note its attachment to the maxilla on the medial wall of the orbit. Carefully remove the medial palpebral ligament and expose the *lacrimal sac* deep to the ligament (Fig. 49.2). The lacrimal sac continues down as the *nasolacrimal duct* which opens into the inferior meatus of the nasal cavity.

Cut through the conjunctiva and the lateral palpebral ligament and detach

the eyeball from the orbit. Cut the eyeball transversely at the equator. In the posterior half, look for the *optic disc* on the *retina*. This is the point of commencement of the optic nerve. Look for the retinal arteries and veins radiating from the optic disc. Lateral to the optic disc is the *macula lutea*, the area for most acute vision. All these structures can be seen during an ophthalmoscopic examination (Fig. 49.3).

In the anterior half of the eyeball study the *lens, ciliary processes* and the *iris* (Fig. 49.4). The circular hole bounded by the iris is the *pupil*. Examine the *cornea,* the *sclera* and the *sclerocorneal junction.* Define the *anterior chamber* which is the space between the cornea and the iris, and the *posterior chamber* between the iris and the lens. The anterior and the posterior chambers communicate through the pupil.

THE EAR

The ear consists of three parts (Fig. 49.5):

- the *external ear,* which collects the sound waves at the ear drum, the *tympanic membrane*
- the *middle ear,* an air-containing space, where the vibrations from the tympanic membrane are transmitted by a chain of three ossicles to the inner ear
- the *inner ear,* a fluid-filled sac containing the sensory receptors for hearing and balance connected to the *vestibulocochlear nerve* (VIII).

Dissection of the middle ear

This is done better on decalcified bone as the petrous part of the temporal bone is hard and difficult to cut in cadaveric specimens.

Make a longitudinal section of the temporal bone along the line shown in Figure 49.6. Examine the lateral half of the section and identify the *tympanic membrane* and the *malleus* and the *incus.* The malleus is attached to the tympanic membrane (Fig. 49.6). On the medial half identify the structures shown in Figure 49.7. Note that anteriorly the *auditory tube* opens into the middle ear and that posteriorly it communicates with the *mastoid antrum* and the *mastoid air cells.* The facial nerve which enters the internal *acoustic meatus* (arrowed in Fig. 49.6) traverses the temporal bone in a bony canal which bulges into the medial wall of the middle ear. Compare your specimen to Figure 49.8 which is a section of a dry temporal bone.

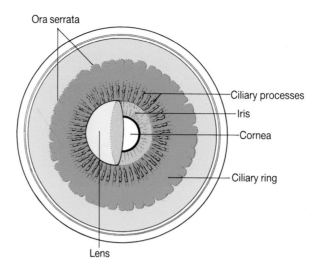

Fig. 49.4 **Ora serrata and lens: posterior view**

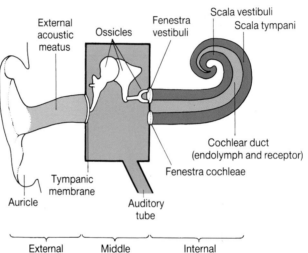

Fig. 49.5 **Design of the ear**

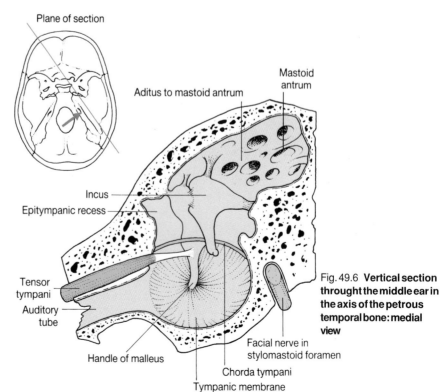

Fig. 49.6 **Vertical section throught the middle ear in the axis of the petrous temporal bone: medial view**

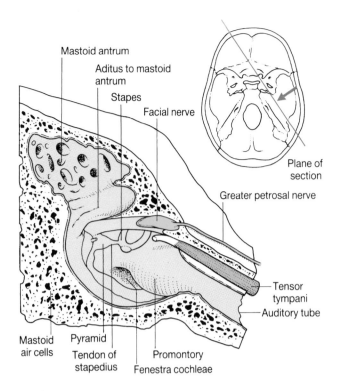

Mastoid antrum

Aditus to mastoid antrum

Stapes

Facial nerve

Plane of section

Greater petrosal nerve

Tensor tympani

Auditory tube

Mastoid air cells

Pyramid

Tendon of stapedius

Promontory

Fenestra cochleae

Fig. 49.7 **Vertical section similar to Figure 48.6.** Here, the medial wall of the middle ear is seen from the lateral side

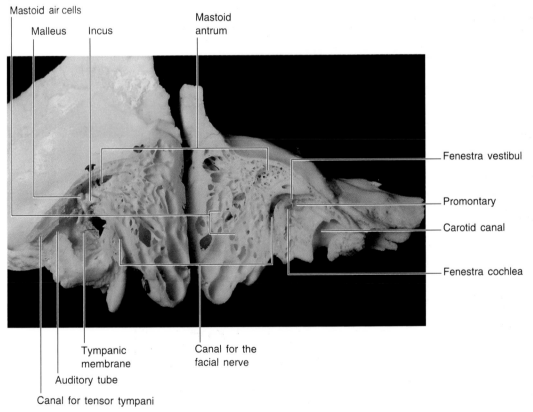

Mastoid air cells

Malleus   Incus

Mastoid antrum

Fenestra vestibul

Promontary

Carotid canal

Fenestra cochlea

Tympanic membrane

Canal for the facial nerve

Auditory tube

Canal for tensor tympani

Fig. 49.8 **Section of right temporal bone**

INDEX

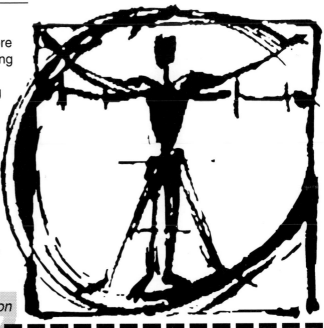

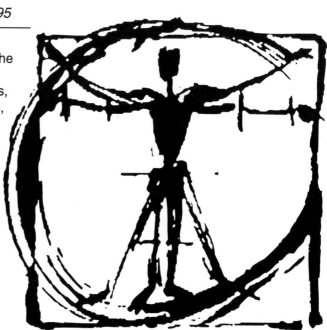